Celiac Disease and Gluten-Free Diet

Edited by Luis Rodrigo

Published in London, United Kingdom

Celiac Disease and Gluten-Free Diet
http://dx.doi.org/10.5772/intechopen.105328
Edited by Luis Rodrigo

Contributors
Karunesh Kumar, Deepika Rustogi, Irati Mendia Azkoaga, Ángel Cebolla, Rahma Al Kindi, Asma Al Salmani, Rahma Al Hadhrami, Maryam Al Maashani, Priscila Farage, Maiara Botosso, Renatta Damasceno, Luis Rodrigo

First published in London, United Kingdom, 2023 by IntechOpen
IntechOpen is the global imprint of INTECHOPEN LIMITED, registered in England and Wales, registration number: 11086078, 5 Princes Gate Court, London, SW7 2QJ, United Kingdom

British Library Cataloguing-in-Publication Data
A catalogue record for this book is available from the British Library

Additional hard and PDF copies can be obtained from orders@intechopen.com

Celiac Disease and Gluten-Free Diet
Edited by Luis Rodrigo
p. cm.
Print ISBN 978-1-83768-870-8
Online ISBN 978-1-83768-871-5
eBook (PDF) ISBN 978-1-83768-872-2

Meet the editor

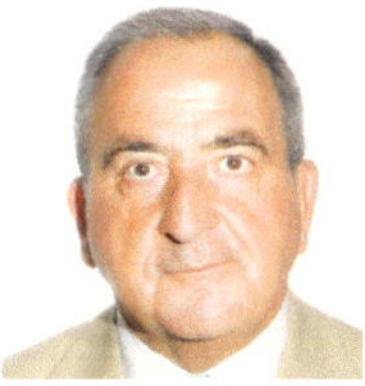

Luis Rodrigo, MD, is a distinguished Professor Emeritus at the University of Oviedo, Spain. With an extensive academic career, he has made significant contributions to the field of medicine. Throughout his professional journey, he has amassed an impressive body of work, including over 500 scientific publications, 20 books, and 58 book chapters. Dr. Rodrigo's expertise in gastroenterology is well recognized. He began his medical specialization in 1972 and went on to hold key positions in the field. In 1976, he became the Chief of Section in Gastroenterology at the University Hospital Central of Asturias (Spain), a role he held until 1988 when he assumed the prestigious position of Chief of Service. His commitment to academic excellence led him to join the University of Oviedo, where he served as a Titular Professor in Medicine from 1983 until 2009. Since 2010, he has held the esteemed position of Full Professor in Medicine at the same institution, and in 2014, he was honored with the title of Emeritus Professor. Dr. Rodrigo's impact extends beyond his own accomplishments. Over the course of 42 years, he has mentored and guided approximately 100 specialists in gastroenterology as part of the National Program of Fellowship, contributing to the development of the next generation of medical professionals. His research contributions are widely recognized both nationally and internationally. He has authored or co-authored 434 scientific papers written in English and 282 in Spanish. Additionally, Dr. Rodrigo has authored 58 chapters in books focused on gastroenterology and has written 20 books exploring various aspects of "Gastroenterological Diseases" as well as other digestive and liver disorders.

Contents

Preface

Celiac disease (CD) is an immune-based systemic disorder caused by the ingestion of gluten and other related proteins that affects genetically susceptible individuals. It is characterized by the presence of a variety of clinical manifestations dependent on gluten ingestion, specific circulating autoantibodies, human leukocyte antigen (HLA), DQ2 (DQ2.5 and/or DQ2.2) and/or haplotypes, and enteropathy.

CD has experienced a notable increase in its prevalence in the last three to four decades, being one of the most frequent genetically transmitted diseases in countries with a predominantly Caucasian population (prevalence 1:100 to 1:250).

Despite the advances in its knowledge and the development and improvement of serological tests, CD continues to be an underdiagnosed entity. This is largely due to the systemic nature of the disease with the involvement of multiple organs and systems. The "classic" pattern of CD is not the most common, especially in adults, where non-specific gastrointestinal symptoms or extra-digestive manifestations of various kinds may be the predominant symptoms.

Some of these patients exhibit low antibody (Ab) titers and low-grade histological lesions. In this context, it should not be surprising that patients take months or years to be diagnosed, or remain undiagnosed for life, partly due to a lack of awareness of the heterogeneity in their patterns of presentation.

The delay or absence of diagnosis can have important consequences for the health and quality of life of those affected. In turn, the recognition of cases, especially in adults, with low-grade histological lesions and negative serology carries the risk of "overdiagnosing" patients whose lesions are actually due to another cause. Therefore, underdiagnosis and overdiagnosis entail the need for an in-depth review of the clinical, serological, genetic, and anatomopathological criteria that make it possible to establish a reliable and trustworthy diagnosis of CD.

A strict gluten-free diet (GFD) leads to the disappearance of symptoms, normalization of serological tests, and resolution of histological lesions in the majority of patients. In addition, indefinite GFD prevents complications and reduces long-term morbidity/mortality.

I want to thank all the participating authors for their excellent and clear contributions. I also want to express my sincere and deep gratitude to the staff at IntechOpen, especially Ms. Ana Cink for her excellent assistance throughout the publication process.

Luis Rodrigo, MD
Professor of Medicine,
Internal Medicine Department,
Oviedo University,
Oviedo, Asturias, Spain

Chapter 1

Introductory Chapter: Celiac Disease – An Overview

Luis Rodrigo

1. Introduction

Celiac disease (CD) is a multisystemic autoimmune-based process, caused by the ingestion of foods containing gluten and related prolamins, which affects genetically susceptible individuals, and is characterized by the presence of a variable combination of various gluten-dependent clinical manifestations, CD-specific antibodies, presence of compatible genetic markers of susceptibility (HLA, DQ2, or DQ8 haplotypes), and enteropathy. The most frequent pathological finding is the presence of chronic inflammation at the small intestine. The estimated average prevalence is around 1%, worldwide, being more frequent in women, with a 2:1 ratio. This definition was updated by the ESPGHAN, European Society for Pediatric Gastroenterology, Hepatology and Nutrition in 2012 [1].

Around 50% of all celiac patients remain undiagnosed for a long time. However, the recognition of other atypical forms of presentation, such as oligo and asymptomatic, combined with greater and better use of the complementary tests available, has made it possible to reveal the existence of different types of CD.

2. Clinical presentations

a. Symptomatic: The symptoms are very diverse, but all patients have serology, histology, and genetic tests compatible with CD.

b. Subclinical: Patients do not show symptoms or signs, although the rest of the diagnostic tests are positive.

c. Latent: These are patients who, at a certain time, while consuming gluten, do not present symptoms and the intestinal mucosa is completely normal.

d. Refractory. This is a very rare form consisting of a lack of response to the gluten-free diet and can be associated with intestinal complications [2].

3. Etiological theories

The cause/s of celiac intolerance are generally unknown, but they are probably related to the presence of one favorable genetic susceptibility to the development of

IntechOpen

gluten intolerance. Thus, various environmental agents have been implicated, such as an increased and continued consumption of foods rich in gluten, as well as probably the presence of triggering viral, bacterial, or parasitic infections.

There is a great overlapping between CD and other autoimmune diseases.

4. Symptomatology

The clinical symptoms are diverse, the most frequent being those of a digestive type such as abdominal distension, nausea, vomiting, diarrhea, abdominal pain, and meteorism, generally accompanied by a decrease in appetite, as well as muscle mass loss, weight, increased tiredness, growth retardation, character changes (irritability, apathy, introversion, sadness, etc.), iron deficiency anemia resistant to treatment, etc. However, in both children and adults, the symptoms may be atypical, or completely absent, making diagnosis difficult [3].

It is estimated that a very high percentage of patients (>75%) are undiagnosed, largely due to the ignorance of primary care physicians, who are the first filter through which celiac people pass. The lack of knowledge about the heterogeneity of the possible symptoms associated with celiac disease in the medical community can cause a significant delay of several years or even a lack of diagnosis. However, the recognition of other atypical and asymptomatic forms of manifestation, combined with the greater and better use of the complementary tests available, has made it possible to reveal the existence of different types of celiac disease.

5. Diagnostic procedures

Diagnosis of celiac disease can be difficult because the symptoms caused by this disease can also appear in many other diseases. Patients with celiac disease usually have elevated serum levels of antibodies against gluten (i.e., anti-gliadin antibodies, anti-transglutaminase, anti-endomysium, and also anti-gliadin deamidated peptide antibodies). If the levels of these antibodies in the blood are elevated then it helps to get a positive diagnosis. The best way to confirm the disease is to perform a duodenoscopy taking several biopsies of the intestinal mucosa to evaluate the degree of inflammatory lesions and the presence or absence of associated villous atrophy. Doubtful cases is useful to perform a flow cytometric study of the duodenal biopsies, in order to classify the lymphocytes subpopulations presented [4].

6. Duodenal biopsies

The confirmation of the diagnosis today is based on the concurrence of clinical suspicion, positive serology, presence of a compatible genetic susceptibility, and findings at the intestinal biopsies compatible with celiac disease.

7. Gluten-free diet

The only treatment for celiac disease is to avoid completely the consumption of foods containing gluten, even in minimal amounts.

Once the gluten-free diet (GFD) is established, the clinical recovery is usually not immediate, and duodenal biopsies can be repeated after 2 years to return to being completely normal [5].

At the beginning of the treatment, in addition to the GFD, dietary supplements of vitamins or minerals can be recommended in some people which show deficiencies and usually, they achieve a faster recovery.

Author details

Luis Rodrigo
School of Medicine, Oviedo University, Oviedo, Spain

*Address all correspondence to: lrodrigosaez@gmail.com

References

[1] Husby S, Koletzko S, Korponay-Szabó IR, Mearin ML, Phillips A, Shamir R, et al. European society for pediatric gastroenterology, hepatology, and nutrition guidelines for the diagnosis of coeliac disease. Journal of Pediatric Gastroenterology and Nutrition. 2012;**54**:136-160

[2] Green PHR, Paski S, Ko CW, Rubio-Tapia A. AGA clinical practice update on management of refractory celiac disease: Expert review. Gastroenterology. 2022;**163**:1461-1469

[3] Ciccocioppo R, Kruzliak P, Cangemi GC, Pohanka M, Betti E, Lauret E, et al. The spectrum of differences between childhood and adulthood celiac disease. Nutrients. 2015;7:8733-8751

[4] Fernández-Bañares F, Carrasco A, García-Puig R, Rosinach M, González C, Alsina M, et al. Intestinal intraepithelial lymphocyte cytometric pattern is more accurate than subepithelial deposits of anti-tissue transglutaminase IgA for the diagnosis of celiac disease in lymphocytic enteritis. PLoS One. 2014;**9**(7):e101249

[5] Sategna-Guidetti C, Grosso SB, Grosso S, Mengozzi G, Aimo G, Zaccaria T, et al. The effects of 1 year gluten withdrawal on bone mass, bone metabolism and nutritional status in newly diagnosed adult coeliac disease patients. Alimentary Pharmacology & Therapeutics. 2000;**14**:35-43

Chapter 2

Extraintestinal Manifestations of Celiac Disease in Children

Karunesh Kumar and Deepika Rustogi

Abstract

Celiac disease can involve any organ system, leading to various non-classical or atypical manifestations. These atypical signs and symptoms have been seen increasingly in the last few decades, both in children and adults, which may or may not involve the gastrointestinal system. This transition from a malabsorptive disorder causing GI symptoms and malnutrition to a more subtle condition causing a variety of extraintestinal manifestations led to newer nomenclature of gastrointestinal and extraintestinal signs and symptoms. Infancy and early childhood onset celiac disease may have a predominance of gastrointestinal manifestations leading to protein energy malnutrition and failure to thrive. The late presentation may have subtle manifestations, and extraintestinal signs and symptoms may be commoner. Short stature, delayed puberty, osteopenia, neuropsychiatric manifestations, iron-deficiency anemia, and elevated liver enzymes are common extraintestinal symptoms. The pathogenesis of extraintestinal manifestations may be due to malabsorption or associated with a systemic autoimmune response. These atypical presentations, especially in the absence of gastrointestinal symptoms and family history, may be missed, leading to a delay in diagnosis and management. A suitable case-finding strategy and liberal use of serological tests may improve the detection rate of CD.

Keywords: celiac disease, gluten-free diet, wheat allergy, atypical celiac, asymptomatic celiac

1. Introduction

Celiac disease (CD) is common in all ages and has various signs and symptoms. These symptoms could be classified as classical (chronic diarrhea and weight loss, etc.) or non-classical (anemia, osteoporosis, neurological disturbances, etc.). Due to atypical manifestations, many CD cases currently escape diagnosis and are exposed to the risk of long-term complications. Infancy and early childhood-onset celiac disease may have a predominance of gastrointestinal manifestations leading to protein energy malnutrition and failure to thrive. Late presentation may have subtle manifestations, and extraintestinal signs and symptoms may be commoner.

Non-classical or atypical symptoms have been increasingly recognized in the last few decades and have become commoner than classical presentation. Due to increasing awareness and serological screening of at-risk groups, non-classical forms are being recognized more yet awareness is lacking [1–3]. Even though this term, typical or atypical, is discouraged but remains in common use, the European Society of Pediatric Gastroenterology Hepatology and Nutrition (ESPGHAN) working group recommends the following nomenclature: gastrointestinal and extraintestinal symptoms and signs [4].

Gastrointestinal manifestations may include nonspecific recurrent abdominal pain, irritable bowel-like symptoms (e.g., recurrent diarrhea), and recurrent aphthous stomatitis. The most frequent extraintestinal presentations include (a) iron deficiency which may or may not be associated with anemia; (b)isolated elevation of liver transaminases (celiac hepatitis) characterized by non-progressive inflammation of liver parenchyma; (c) short stature and delayed puberty. CD is one of the commonest causes of short stature and is characterized by delayed bone age, either normal or blunted growth hormone response to stimulatory tests and low levels of insulin-like growth factor-1 [5]; (d) chronic fatigue; (e) behavioral disturbances, such as irritability, and impaired school performance. Detailed list is mentioned in **Table 1**. Extraintestinal symptoms occur at similar rates in children and in adults: 60 and 62%, respectively [7]. However, clinical manifestations and rate of improvement differ in the two age groups. In children, short stature, fatigue, and headache appear to be the most common, while iron-deficiency anemia is the predominant manifestation in adults. Children respond faster to GFD in the resolution of symptoms than in adults [7, 8]. While some of the extraintestinal manifestations, such as weight loss, fatigue, short stature, and delayed

Extraintestinal symptoms	Percentage of total no. children/ adolescents with CD
• Weight loss, failure-to-thrive, stunted growth/short stature.	19–31
• Delayed puberty and amenorrhea	11–20
• Irritability and chronic fatigue	10–14, 7
• Chronic iron-deficiency anemia	3–16
• Joint and musculoskeletal disorders	5–10
• Bone diseases—decreased bone mineralization and repetitive fractures	75 46
• Recurrent aphthous stomatitis	4
• Dermatitis herpetiformis-type rash	5
• Dental enamel defects	9–14
• Abnormal liver biochemistry	1
• Alopecia areata	0.1–7.4
• Neuropathy	18
• Headache and migraine	0.7–2
• Idiopathic seizures	
• Depression and psychiatric disorders	
• Vitamin deficiency	

Table 1.
Extraintestinal symptoms and their prevalence [4, 6].

puberty, can be attributed to nutritional deficiencies and their metabolic consequences, others follow different and often poorly understood pathways.

2. Diagnosis

It is crucial to diagnose CD not only in children with obvious gastrointestinal symptoms but also in children with a less clear clinical picture because the disease may have negative health consequences. Children with extraintestinal manifestations may present to a different speciality, which sometimes makes diagnosis difficult because of unfamiliarity with the disease. This undiagnosed proportion can be as high as 85–90% [9, 10]. Because atypical symptoms may be considerably more common than classic symptoms, the ESPGHAN working group decided to use the following nomenclature: gastrointestinal symptoms and signs (e.g., chronic diarrhea) and extraintestinal symptoms and signs (e.g., anemia, neuropathy, decreased bone density, increased risk of fractures) [4]. Based on this, they recommended CD testing in children and adolescents with the following otherwise unexplained symptoms and signs: chronic abdominal pain, cramping or distension, chronic or intermittent diarrhea, growth failure, iron-deficiency anemia, nausea or vomiting, chronic constipation not responding to usual treatment, weight loss, chronic fatigue, short stature, delayed puberty, amenorrhea, recurrent aphthous stomatitis (mouth ulcers), dermatitis herpetiformis-type rash, repetitive fractures/osteopenia/osteoporosis, and unexplained abnormal liver biochemistry [4, 6].

3. Underlying pathophysiology

Two mechanisms play crucial roles in the pathogenesis of extraintestinal manifestations: proximal bowel mucosal damage and the autoimmune response. However, many aspects of pathogenesis remain unclear. Many of the extraintestinal manifestations correlate with the extent of intestinal damage but may not be true for all. Anemia, stunted growth, and osteopenia are some examples correlating with the extent of damage and consequent malabsorption. Autoimmune phenomenon plays a role in some extraintestinal manifestations, but correlation or justification may not be straightforward. Tissue transglutaminase 2 (TG2) is the main, but not the only autoantigen involved in CD. IgA deposits co-localize with TG2 in the liver, lymph nodes, muscle, thyroid, bone, and brain indicating that the autoantibodies, probably originated in the gut, can access TG2 throughout the body and cause pathogenic effects. Other autoantibodies which can have possible roles in the pathogenesis of extraintestinal manifestations in CD are tissue transglutaminase 3 (TG3) and tissue transglutaminase 6 (TG6). The TG3 is mainly expressed in the epidermis, and its presence is used as a diagnostic test for DH. They are also present in areas away from the skin lesions, suggesting that other factors might have a role. The TG6 is mainly expressed in the neurons, and an association between neurological symptoms and the presence of anti-TG6 antibodies has been postulated. Again, their presence in asymptomatic patients may suggest other unknown mechanisms may have a role. Specificity of these autoantibodies and the gluten-dependence of their production have not been definitely proven [11]. Antibodies to gangliosides have been reported in immune-mediated peripheral neuropathies and in patients with neurological symptoms, their titers reduced on GFD [12] (**Table 2**).

Extraintestinal symptoms	Possible underlying pathogenic mechanism
Delayed puberty and amenorrhea	Malnutrition, hypothalamic-pituitary dysfunction, and immune dysfunction
Weight loss, failure-to-thrive, stunted growth/short stature	Malnutrition, hypothalamic-pituitary dysfunction, and vitamin deficiency
Chronic iron-deficiency anemia	Iron, folate, vitamin B12, or pyridoxine deficiency
Dermatitis herpetiformis-type rash	Epidermal (type 3) TG autoimmunity
Irritability and chronic fatigue	Generalized muscle atrophy, hypokalemia
Abnormal liver biochemistry	Celiac hepatitis, autoimmune hepatitis
Neuropathy	Deficiencies of vitamin B12 and thiamine; immune-based neurologic dysfunction
Idiopathic seizures	unknown
Neuro-psychiatric manifestation	Immune-based neurologic dysfunction Cerebellar and posterior column damage
Recurrent aphthous stomatitis	Unknown
Decreased bone mineralization (osteopenia/osteoporosis) and repetitive fractures	Malabsorption of calcium and vitamin D, secondary hyperparathyroidism, and chronic inflammation
Dental enamel defects	Vitamin D and calcium malabsorption

Table 2.
Extraintestinal manifestations and their underlying pathophysiology [13].

4. Extraintestinal manifestations

4.1 Weight loss, failure-to-thrive, and stunted growth/short stature

Short stature can be an isolated initial presentation, it is one of the commonest extraintestinal manifestations of CD in children, and 10 to 40% will have short stature at the time of diagnosis [7]. Severe growth failure, along with severe disease onset, has been commonly seen in younger children [14]. CD can be found in up to 10% of children undergoing evaluation for short stature [15], which is between 19 and 59% of all non-endocrinological causes [16, 17]. Recently, a meta-analysis found one in 14 patients with all-cause short stature and one in nine patients with idiopathic short stature to have a biopsy-confirmed CD [18]. Such children respond well and show catch-up growth to GFD if the diagnosis has been made well before puberty [7].

4.2 Delayed puberty and amenorrhea

The prevalence of delayed puberty is seen in up to 20% of children with celiac disease [19]. This could be because of hypogonadism or hormonal resistance [20]. Hormonal resistance can develop due to antibodies against hormones, their receptors, or endocrine organs. Nutrition may also play a role. These patients respond very well to GFD, and puberty occurs within 6–8 months.

4.3 Chronic iron-deficiency anemia

Iron-deficiency anemia (IDA) is adults' most common extraintestinal manifestation. Delay in diagnosis in adults could be one of the reasons for higher prevalence.

Prevalence in children has been found to be around 15% [7, 8]. It can be the sole manifestation or presenting feature of CD, especially in older children and adolescents. Iron deficiency may or may not be associated with anemia. In the ProCeDE study, the cohort of children diagnosed based on symptoms, iron-deficiency anemia was reported in 17% [21]. A large pediatric population-based study in Germany found no significant differences between TGA-IgA positive children compared with negatives. Still, serum ferritin was significantly lower in the seropositive group, indicating lower iron stores [22]. A different study from the same region found CD in 6 (4.4%) IDA patients without gastrointestinal symptoms, but they found zero cases in 223 healthy asymptomatic children without anemia [23].

Anemia, most commonly IDA, in CD children can result from several different, and sometimes combined, causes [24]. IDA severity co-relates with the disease severity (histological and serological) and could be a manifestation of malabsorption due to damage in the proximal small bowel [25, 26]. However, even when asymptomatic, CD can lead to IDA [27]. Iron absorption occurs in the proximal small bowel, the area most commonly involved in CD, which explains the IDA. Vit B12 and folate deficiency can also contribute to the pathogenesis of anemia. But anemia in potential celiac, in the absence of histopathological changes, suggests the role of some other mechanism as well. Majority of (up to 84%) children with CD presenting with mild anemia on strict GFD and iron supplementation replenish their iron stores by 12–24 months [7, 25].

4.4 Joint and musculoskeletal disorders

Though rare, joint involvement has been reported in children and adults with CD [28]. It can be in the form of arthralgia, arthritis (non-erosive), and myopathy, which may be silent in the initial stages of the disease. Joint and musculoskeletal involvement may be because of other associated underlying autoimmune conditions, which are relatively common in children with CD and should be ruled out first before attributing it to CD. Pathophysiology of musculoskeletal involvement in CD is not very well understood, and even response to GFD is not consistent [29]. Patients with unexplained arthralgia/arthritis should be tested for underlying CD once other autoimmune musculoskeletal conditions have been ruled out [30].

4.5 Decreased bone mineralization (osteopenia/osteoporosis), repetitive fractures

Approximately 75% of pediatric patients have osteopenia (low bone mineral density), and 10–30% have osteoporosis (bone brittleness) [31]. Decreased bone mineralization can be due to a combination of intestinal malabsorption (the majority of calcium and vitamin D gets absorbed from the proximal small intestine, which is damaged in a patient with CD) and chronic inflammation. Low level of vitamin D can lead to a high level of parathyroid, which is a common finding in such patients. Hyperparathyroidism and other intermediate metabolites lead to higher bone turnover, causing osteopenia and osteoporosis. Higher serum OPG, telopeptide, and lower serum pro-peptide have been found in these patients, pointing again toward an increased bone turnover [32]. Growing trabecular bones are commonly involved. Osteopenia can even be found in the early stages of CD hence the emphasis on early detection and treatment. Osteopenia in children with CD responds very well to the GFD. Even adult patients too can improve their bone mineral density after some years on GFD, but the response is not as robust [33]. Vitamin D and calcium supplementation can hasten the recovery in such children; hence, adequate supplementation should be ensured in newly diagnosed CD children.

4.6 Oral manifestations and recurrent aphthous stomatitis

Geographical tongue and aphthous ulcers are common oral manifestations in children with CD. Lichen planus, cheilosis, atrophic glossitis, and glossodinia are other common manifestations which may or may not be specific to CD. Children with geographical tongue have more prevalence of CD in comparison with the general population [34]. Aphthous ulcers are a non-specific occurrence in CD and can be found in other autoimmune or medical conditions like IBD and Behcet's disease. The underlying pathogenic mechanism is not very clear and may have some relation with malabsorption, and changes in the normal oral flora and ecosystem may be contributory. Such lesions respond very well to GFD, and they remit completely on GFD.

In a case-control study, 50 CD cases and 50 controls were assessed, and the prevalence of aphthous ulcers was 62% and 13%, respectively [35]. In the same study, delayed dental eruption was observed in 38% and 11% and specific enamel defects in 48% and 0%, respectively [35]. An Iranian study among teenagers and adults reported a prevalence of CD in 2.8% of children with recurrent aphthae and was significantly higher than the general population [36].

4.7 Dermatitis herpetiformis-type rash

DH affects primarily older children and adults. In contrast to CD, the annual incidence of DH has been decreasing probably because of the diagnosis of even silent and asymptomatic patients. It may suggest that subclinical CD may predispose to DH. Gastrointestinal symptoms are rare in patients with DH, but enteropathy can be documented in up to 72% of the patients [37]. DH manifests as bilateral, symmetrical blisters with pruritus affecting extensor surfaces followed by shoulders, buttocks, sacral region, and face. These lesions may be preceded by itching and burning sensation followed by erosions, excoriations, and hyperpigmentation. DH is considered the skin manifestation typical of celiac disease as similar antibodies are at play, which leads to intestinal changes [38]. Epidermal transglutaminase (TG3) acts as an autoantigen against which patient develops an antibody which gets deposited in the skin layer. Characteristic granular IgA deposits can be demonstrated by direct immunofluorescence microscopy in the biopsy of the adjacent unaffected skin at the dermo-epidermal junction [39]. Strict GFD is very effective with 100% resolution, but in the initial phase, dapsone or other drugs can be used.

4.8 Dental enamel defects

Dental enamel hypoplasia is a common occurrence in children, and prevalence ranges between 10% and 97% in various studies. Still, prevalence has been decreasing in recent studies suggesting a less severe presentation of the disease nowadays [40]. Nutritional deficiency due to malabsorption during the period of enamel formation (<7 years), and immunological disturbances lead to the defect. Deciduous teeth (incisors and molars) are more frequently involved in a symmetrical way. The enamel defects manifest as pitting or grooving on the surface or sometimes with complete loss of enamel. They can also include discoloration and structural changes on the surface. These changes improve once nutritional and immunological disturbances are restored. Improvement will occur in primary teeth, but the same may not be valid for permanent teeth, even on strict GFD. These enamel defects, like other extraintestinal manifestations, may or may not have other symptoms and hence can be a useful clinical screening tool [41].

4.9 Elevation of transaminases

Liver enzymes may be deranged in children with CD, a most common hepatic manifestation of CD, which could be related to the disease itself (idiopathic or known as celiac hepatitis) or due to associated autoimmune hepatitis. Celiac hepatitis is seen in about one-third of children with CD [42]. On the contrary, CD may be found in 12% of children with mild unexplained elevated transaminases [42]. Extent of involvement usually correlates with overall disease severity (histopathological and serological). Duodenal damage may expose the liver to hepatotoxins because of the increased permeability, and autoimmune factors may also play a role suggested by the deposition of CD antibodies in the liver [43, 44]. Liver involvement is usually mild and reversible and rarely causes liver failure [45]. When a child presents with deranged liver function and coagulopathy, underlying malabsorption needs to be considered and treated with supplementing Vitamin K. Good compliance with GFD leads to normalization of the liver transaminases levels in up to 95% within 1–2 years [46]. The same is not true if the liver involvement is because of another concomitant autoimmune liver disease.

4.10 Alopecia areata

Alopecia areata is characterized by a patchy hair loss on the scalp, a common form of hair loss in children. It is believed to be an autoimmune condition and is common in CD children [47]. It can occur in the absence of GI signs and symptoms but, once diagnosed, shows an excellent response to the GFD.

4.11 Headache, migraine, idiopathic seizures, depression, and psychiatric disorders

Neurological symptoms are more common in children with CD than controls [48]. Headache is the most common neurological symptom (in 18%) and responds well to the exclusion of gluten from the diet [49, 50]. Other neurological symptoms are peripheral neuropathy and seizures, which also tend to improve with GFD [48, 51]. Anti-ganglioside antibodies, along with nutritional deficiencies, like Vitamin B12, E, and D, may play a role in neuropathy. These manifestations may be present in children in the absence of enteropathy, suggesting that other mechanisms like a cross-reaction between anti-gliadin antibodies and synapsin might be responsible. Epilepsy's prevalence is higher, though some studies did not find a significant difference in the prevalence, in CD children, and the difference remains uncertain. The seizures are generalized tonic-clonic, but partial and occasionally absence seizures are also seen [52]. GFD helps control frequency of seizure episodes, especially those poorly controlled despite antileptic medications. Epilepsy associated with occipital calcification has been reported in children with CD [53]. A patient with epilepsy disorder without a clear etiology should be considered for CD screening as their seizure control will be better on GFD. Ataxia, a neurological manifestation of CD, tends to manifest predominantly in adult patients. The presence of anti-TG6 antibodies against the cerebellar cells might play a pathogenic role. These autoantibodies can also be found in children without neurological disorders, suggesting some other unknown mechanism.

Psychiatric issues like anxiety, hallucinations, and depression are common in adolescents and may persist into adult life, and interestingly, they respond to GFD [54, 55]. An increased suicide tendency in CD patients has also been observed [56].

4.12 Vitamin deficiency

Vitamin D deficiency is the most common deficiency seen in children with CD, and its testing is recommended at diagnosis so that adequate supplementation can be given. Vitamin D deficiency can lead to hyperparathyroidism and subsequent osteopenia. Other vitamin levels can also be diminished in CD due to malabsorption and manifest in different ways, as discussed in other sections.

5. Peri-natal and post-natal manifestations

Over the last three decades, several reports, mostly retrospective, have examined the potential impact of undiagnosed celiac disease on pregnancy and fetal outcomes. Asymptomatic and undiagnosed celiac disease has been associated with various gynecological, obstetric, and fetal complications with conflicting results, particularly unexplained infertility, miscarriages, fetal growth restriction, low birth weight, and preterm birth [57–60].

The association between untreated maternal celiac disease and intrauterine growth restriction (IUGR) and small for gestational age (SGA) has been highly significant in most scientific reports. The odds ratio from a large population-based Danish cohort study was 1.31 (CI 1.06–1.63) and OR 1.62 (CI 1.22–2.15) in a similar Swedish study [61]. Evidence in favor of the normalization of most of these complications with a gluten-free diet appears reassuring, though the literature is limited [7, 59, 61, 62]. There are some reports concerning the effect of paternal celiac disease on preterm birth and birth weight. However, further research is needed to confirm the findings [63, 64]. We could not find data on the impact of undiagnosed maternal disease on neonates and infants.

6. Treatment

GFD is the only effective therapy available; none of the pharmacological alternatives is effective and can replace GFD [65]. Recovery from GFD is faster in children and can lead to complete remission of extraintestinal manifestations [7]. Starting GFD as soon as possible is essential and will have a good prognosis. This is especially true for bone diseases or short stature.

Nevertheless, sometimes more than the diet is needed, vitamins and minerals need supplementation. Anemia may need iron supplementation, vitamin D deficiency needs supplementation with Vitamin D and calcium, and DH may require medical therapy in the initial days. Compliance is an issue, especially in adolescents, affected with the highest prevalence of extraintestinal manifestations and complications [59]. Compliance needs to be ascertained, especially if there is no improvement in the symptoms. If there is no improvement despite compliance, other diagnoses or pathogenic mechanisms should be investigated, for instance, growth hormone deficiency in children with short stature and hematological disorders in children with anemia.

DOI: http://dx.doi.org/10.5772/intechopen.110370

7. Conclusion

Extraintestinal manifestations are more common in CD in children and often get overlooked because of a lack of awareness. These atypical manifestations make diagnosis difficult, which leads to delay in diagnosis. With easily available efficient screening serological tools, diagnosis can be straightforward, but awareness over the multispecialty levels (hematologists, neurologists, rheumatologists, and endocrinologists) needs to be increased. An early diagnosis is vital to prevent long-term complications, especially those that are no more correctable after a certain age (e.g., osteopenia and short stature).

Acknowledgements

No funding received.

Conflict of interest

The authors declare no conflict of interest.

Appendices and nomenclature

CD	celiac disease
TG	transglutaminase
DH	dermatitis herpetiformis
GFD	gluten-free diet
TGA IgA	transglutaminase antibody IgA
IDA	iron-deficiency anemia
ESPGHAN	European society of pediatric gastroenterology hepatology and nutrition

Author details

Karunesh Kumar[1*] and Deepika Rustogi[2]

1 Indraprastha Apollo Hospitals, New Delhi, India

2 Yashoda Super Specialty Hospital, Kaushambi, Ghaziabad, India

*Address all correspondence to: karuneshgastro@gmail.com

References

[1] Fasano A, Catassi C. Current approaches to diagnosis and treatment of celiac disease: An evolving spectrum. Gastroenterology. 2001;**120**(3):636-651

[2] Fasano A, Araya M, Bhatnagar S, Cameron D, Catassi C, Dirks M, et al. Federation of International Societies of Pediatric Gastroenterology, Hepatology, and Nutrition consensus report on celiac disease. Journal of Pediatric Gastroenterology and Nutrition. 2008;**47**(2):214-219

[3] Bai JC, Fried M, Corazza GR, Schuppan D, Farthing M, Catassi C, et al. World Gastroenterology Organisation global guidelines on celiac disease. Journal of Clinical Gastroenterology. 2013;**47**(2):121-126

[4] Husby S, Koletzko S, Korponay-Szabó IR, Mearin ML, Phillips A, Shamir R, et al. European Society for Pediatric Gastroenterology, Hepatology, and Nutrition guidelines for the diagnosis of coeliac disease. Journal of Pediatric Gastroenterology and Nutrition. 2012;**54**(1):136-160

[5] Catassi C, Fasano A. Celiac disease as a cause of growth retardation in childhood. Current Opinion in Pediatrics. 2004;**16**(4):445-449

[6] Husby S, Koletzko S, Korponay -Szabó I, Kurppa K, Mearin ML, Ribes-Koninckx C, et al. European Society Paediatric Gastroenterology, Hepatology and Nutrition Guidelines for Diagnosing Coeliac Disease 2020. Journal of Pediatric Gastroenterology and Nutrition. 2020;**70**(1):141-156

[7] Jericho H, Sansotta N, Guandalini S. Extraintestinal manifestations of celiac disease: Effectiveness of the gluten-free diet. Journal of Pediatric Gastroenterology and Nutrition. 2017;**65**(1):75-79

[8] Nurminen S, Kivelä L, Huhtala H, Kaukinen K, Kurppa K. Extraintestinal manifestations were common in children with coeliac disease and were more prevalent in patients with more severe clinical and histological presentation. Acta Paediatrica. 2019;**108**(4):681-687

[9] Riznik P, De Leo L, Dolinsek J, Gyimesi J, Klemenak M, Koletzko B, et al. Diagnostic delays in children with coeliac disease in the central European region. Journal of Pediatric Gastroenterology and Nutrition. 2019;**69**(4):443-448

[10] Choung RS, Larson SA, Khaleghi S, Rubio-Tapia A, Ovsyannikova IG, King KS, et al. Prevalence and morbidity of undiagnosed celiac disease from a community-based study. Gastroenterology. 2017;**152**(4):830-839.e5

[11] Mulder CJJ, Rouvroye MD, van Dam AM. Transglutaminase 6 antibodies are not yet mainstream in neuro-coeliac disease. Digestive and Liver Disease. 2018;**50**(1):96-97

[12] Volta U, De Giorgio R, Granito A, Stanghellini V, Barbara G, Avoni P, et al. Anti-ganglioside antibodies in coeliac disease with neurological disorders. Digestive and Liver Disease. 2006;**38**(3):183-187

[13] Nardecchia S, Auricchio R, Discepolo V, Troncone R. Extra-intestinal manifestations of coeliac disease in children: Clinical features and mechanisms. Frontiers in Pediatrics. 2019;7:56

[14] Nurminen S, Kivelä L, Taavela J, Huhtala H, Mäki M, Kaukinen K, et al.

Factors associated with growth disturbance at celiac disease diagnosis in children: A retrospective cohort study. BMC Gastroenterology. 2015;**15**(1):125

[15] Gokce S, Arslantas E. Changing face and clinical features of celiac disease in children: Celiac disease in children. Pediatrics International. 2015;**57**(1):107-112

[16] Saari A, Harju S, Mäkitie O, Saha MT, Dunkel L, Sankilampi U. Systematic growth monitoring for the early detection of celiac disease in children. JAMA Pediatrics. 2015;**169**(3):e1525

[17] Singh P, Sharma PK, Agnihotri A, Jyotsna VP, Das P, Gupta SD, et al. Coeliac disease in patients with short stature: A tertiary care Centre experience. National Medical Journal of India. 2015;**28**(4):176-180

[18] Singh AD, Singh P, Farooqui N, Strand T, Ahuja V, Makharia GK. Prevalence of celiac disease in patients with short stature: A systematic review and meta-analysis. Journal of Gastroenterology and Hepatology. 2021;**36**(1):44-54

[19] Philip R, Patidar P, Saran S, Agarwal P, Arya T, Gupta K. Endocrine manifestations of celiac disease. Indian Journal of Endocrinology Metabolism. 2012;**16**(8):506

[20] Bona G, Marinello D, Oderda G. Mechanisms of abnormal puberty in coeliac disease. Hormone Research in Pædiatrics. 2002;**57**(Suppl. 2):63-65

[21] Werkstetter KJ, Korponay-Szabó IR, Popp A, Villanacci V, Salemme M, Heilig G, et al. Accuracy in diagnosis of celiac disease without biopsies in clinical practice. Gastroenterology. 2017;**153**(4):924-935

[22] Laass MW, Schmitz R, Uhlig HH, Zimmer KP, Thamm M, Koletzko S. The prevalence of celiac disease in children and adolescents in Germany. Deutsches Ärzteblatt International. 17 Aug 2015;**112**(33-34):553-560. DOI: 10.3238/arztebl.2015.0553. PMID: 26356552; PMCID: PMC4570960

[23] Kalayci AG, Kanber Y, Birinci A, Yildiz L, Albayrak D. The prevalence of coeliac disease as detected by screening in children with iron deficiency anaemia: Coeliac disease in children with anaemia. Acta Paediatrica. 2007;**94**(6):678-681

[24] Harper JW, Holleran SF, Ramakrishnan R, Bhagat G, Green PHR. Anemia in celiac disease is multifactorial in etiology. American Journal of Hematology. 2007;**82**(11):996-1000

[25] Rajalahti T, Repo M, Kivelä L, Huhtala H, Mäki M, Kaukinen K, et al. Anemia in Pediatric celiac disease: Association with clinical and histological features and response to gluten-free diet. Journal of Pediatric Gastroenterology and Nutrition. 2017;**64**(1):e1-e6

[26] Zanini B, Caselani F, Magni A, Turini D, Ferraresi A, Lanzarotto F, et al. Celiac disease with mild enteropathy is not mild disease. Clinical Gastroenterology and Hepatology. 2013;**11**(3):253-258

[27] Bottaro G, Cataldo F, Rotolo N, Spina M, Corazza GR. The clinical pattern of subclinical/silent celiac disease: An analysis on 1026 consecutive cases figure 1. The American Journal of Gastroenterology. 1999;**94**(3):691-696

[28] Dos Santos S, Lioté F. Osteoarticular manifestations of celiac disease and non-celiac gluten hypersensitivity. Joint, Bone, Spine. 2017;**84**(3):263-266

[29] Iqbal T, Zaidi MA, Wells GA, Karsh J. Celiac disease arthropathy and

autoimmunity study: Celiac disease arthropathy & autoimmunity. Journal of Gastroenterology and Hepatology. 2013;**28**(1):99-105

[30] Sherman Y, Karanicolas R, DiMarco B, Pan N, Adams AB, Barinstein LV, et al. Unrecognized celiac disease in children presenting for rheumatology evaluation. Pediatrics. 2015;**136**(1):e68-e75

[31] Pantaleoni S, Luchino M, Adriani A, Pellicano R, Stradella D, Ribaldone DG, et al. Bone mineral density at diagnosis of celiac disease and after 1 year of gluten-free diet. Scientific World Journal. 2014;**2014**:1-6

[32] Di Stefano M, Bergonzi M, Benedetti I, De Amici M, Torre C, Brondino N, et al. Alterations of inflammatory and matrix production indices in celiac disease with low bone mass on long-term gluten-free diet. Journal of Clinical Gastroenterology. 2019;**53**(6):e221-e226

[33] Hære P, Høie O, Lundin KEA, Haugeberg G. No major reduction in bone mineral density after long-term treatment of patients with celiac disease. European Journal of Internal Medicine. 2019;**68**:23-29

[34] Cigic L, Galic T, Kero D, Simunic M, Medvedec Mikic I, Kalibovic Govorko D, et al. The prevalence of celiac disease in patients with geographic tongue. Journal of Oral Pathology & Medicine. 2016;**45**(10):791-796

[35] Bramanti E, Cicciù M, Matacena G, Costa S, Magazzù G. Clinical evaluation of specific Oral manifestations in Pediatric patients with ascertained versus potential coeliac disease: A cross-sectional study. Gastroenterology Research and Practice. 2014;**2014**:1-9

[36] Shakeri R, Zamani F, Sotoudehmanesh R, Amiri A, Mohamadnejad M, Davatchi F, et al. Gluten sensitivity enteropathy in patients with recurrent aphthous stomatitis. BMC Gastroenterology. 2009;**9**(1):44

[37] Mansikka E, Hervonen K, Kaukinen K, Collin P, Huhtala H, Reunala T, et al. Prognosis of dermatitis Herpetiformis patients with and without villous atrophy at diagnosis. Nutrients. 2018;**10**(5):641

[38] Reunala T, Salmi T, Hervonen K, Kaukinen K, Collin P. Dermatitis Herpetiformis: A common extraintestinal manifestation of coeliac disease. Nutrients. 2018;**10**(5):602

[39] Zone JJ, Meyer LJ, Petersen MJ. Deposition of granular IgA relative to clinical lesions in dermatitis herpetiformis. Archives of Dermatology. 1996;**132**(8):912-918

[40] Souto-Souza D, da Consolação Soares ME, Rezende VS, de Lacerda Dantas PC, Galvão EL, Falci SGM. Association between developmental defects of enamel and celiac disease: A meta-analysis. Archives of Oral Biology. 2018;**87**:180-190

[41] Martelossi S, Zanatta E, Santo E, Clarich P, Radovich P, Ventura A. Dental enamel defects and screening for coeliac disease. Acta Paediatrica. 1996;**85**(s412):47-48

[42] Vajro P, Paolella G, Maggiore G, Giordano G. Pediatric celiac disease, cryptogenic Hypertransaminasemia, and autoimmune hepatitis. Journal of Pediatric Gastroenterology and Nutrition. 2013;**56**(6):663-670

[43] Anania C, Luca ED, Castro GD, Chiesa C, Pacifico L. Liver involvement in pediatric celiac disease. World Journal of Gastroenterology. 2015;**21**(19):5813-5822

[44] Korponay-Szabo IR. In vivo targeting of intestinal and extraintestinal transglutaminase 2 by coeliac autoantibodies. Gut. 2004;**53**(5):641-648

[45] Kaukinen K, Halme L, Collin P, Färkkilä M, Mäki M, Vehmanen P, et al. Celiac disease in patients with severe liver disease: Gluten-free diet may reverse hepatic failure. Gastroenterology. 2002;**122**(4):881-888

[46] Lee GJ, Boyle B, Ediger T, Hill I. Hypertransaminasemia in newly diagnosed Pediatric patients with celiac disease. Journal of Pediatric Gastroenterology and Nutrition. 2016;**63**(3):340-343

[47] Ertekin V, Tosun M, Erdem T. Screening of celiac disease in children with alopecia areata. Indian Journal of Dermatology. 2014;**59**(3):317

[48] Mearns E, Taylor A, Thomas Craig K, Puglielli S, Leffler D, Sanders D, et al. Neurological manifestations of neuropathy and Ataxia in celiac disease: A systematic review. Nutrients. 2019;**11**(2):380

[49] Dimitrova AK, Ungaro RC, Lebwohl B, Lewis SK, Tennyson CA, Green MW, et al. Prevalence of migraine in patients with celiac disease and inflammatory bowel disease. Headache Journal of Head and Face Pain. 2013;**53**(2):344-355

[50] Nenna R, Petrarca L, Verdecchia P, Florio M, Pietropaoli N, Mastrogiorgio G, et al. Celiac disease in a large cohort of children and adolescents with recurrent headache: A retrospective study. Digestive and Liver Disease. 2016;**48**(5):495-498

[51] Bashiri H, Afshari D, Babaei N, Ghadami MR. Celiac disease and epilepsy: The effect of gluten-free diet on seizure control. Advances in Clinical and Experimental Medicine. 2016;**25**(4):751-754

[52] Canova C, Ludvigsson JF, Barbiellini Amidei C, Zanier L, Zingone F. The risk of epilepsy in children with celiac disease: A population-based cohort study. European Journal of Neurology. 2020;**27**(6):1089-1095

[53] Zelnik N, Pacht A, Obeid R, Lerner A. Range of neurologic disorders in patients with celiac disease. Pediatrics. 2004;**113**(6):1672-1676

[54] Lebwohl B, Haggård L, Emilsson L, Söderling J, Roelstraete B, Butwicka A, et al. Psychiatric disorders in patients with a diagnosis of celiac disease during childhood from 1973 to 2016. Clinical Gastroenterology and Hepatology. 2021;**19**(10):2093-2101

[55] Simsek S, Baysoy G, Gencoglan S, Uluca U. Effects of gluten-free diet on quality of life and depression in children with celiac disease. Journal of Pediatric Gastroenterology and Nutrition. 2015;**61**(3):303-306

[56] Ludvigsson JF, Sellgren C, Runeson B, Långström N, Lichtenstein P. Increased suicide risk in coeliac disease—A Swedish nationwide cohort study. Digestive and Liver Disease. 2011;**43**(8):616-622

[57] Martinelli P. Coeliac disease and unfavourable outcome of pregnancy. Gut. 2000;**46**(3):332-335

[58] Gasbarrini A, Torre ES, Trivellini C, De Carolis S, Caruso A, Gasbarrini G. Recurrent spontaneous abortion and intrauterine fetal growth retardation as symptoms of coeliac disease. The Lancet. 2000;**356**(9227):399-400

[59] Ludvigsson J, Montgomery S, Ekbom A. Celiac disease and risk of

adverse Fetal outcome: A population-based cohort study. Gastroenterology. 2005;**129**(2):454-463

[60] Salvatore S, Finazzi S, Radaelli G, Lotzniker M, Zuccotti GV. Prevalence of undiagnosed celiac disease in the parents of preterm and/or small for gestational age infants. The American Journal of Gastroenterology. 2007;**102**(1):168-173

[61] Khashan AS, Henriksen TB, Mortensen PB, McNamee R, McCarthy FP, Pedersen MG, et al. The impact of maternal celiac disease on birthweight and preterm birth: A Danish population-based cohort study. Human Reproduction. 2010;**25**(2):528-534

[62] Tursi A, Giorgetti G, Brandimarte G, Elisei W. Effect of gluten-free diet on pregnancy outcome in celiac disease patients with recurrent miscarriages. Digestive Diseases and Sciences. 2008;**53**(11):2925-2928

[63] Ludvigsson JF, Montgomery SM, Ekbom A. Coeliac disease in the father and risk of adverse pregnancy outcome: A population-based cohort study. Scandinavian Journal of Gastroenterology. 2006;**41**(2):178-185

[64] Khashan AS, Kenny LC, McNamee R, Mortensen PB, Pedersen MG, McCarthy FP, et al. Undiagnosed coeliac disease in a father does not influence birthweight and preterm birth: Paternal coeliac and disease pregnancy outcome. Paediatric and Perinatal Epidemiology. 2010;**24**(4):363-369

[65] Ludvigsson JF, Ciacci C, Green PH, Kaukinen K, Korponay-Szabo IR, Kurppa K, et al. Outcome measures in coeliac disease trials: The Tampere recommendations. Gut. 2018;**67**(8):1410-1424

Chapter 3

Current Trends in the GFD Follow-Up

Irati Mendia Azkoaga and Ángel Cebolla

Abstract

A poor adherence to a gluten-free diet (GFD) have a negative impact on people with celiac disease (CD). However, committing to a gluten-free lifelong carries social and economic burden and, a high degree of knowledge, motivation and a continuous effort. It is essential that the patient understands its disease, how to perform a GFD and the consequences that entail if the patient is not followed in the long term. However, a large percentage of patients does not still achieve a complete mucosal healing, likely due to a poor adherence to the GFD. We describe the current tools for the control of adherence to a GFD, with a special focus on the detection of gluten immunogenic peptides (GIP) in feces and urine, as GIP detection allows direct evidence that the gluten that has been ingested. GIP are becoming useful biomarkers for this aim. Here, we summarize the current information about the main applications and limitations of the use of the GIP determinations in the follow up of celiac disease.

Keywords: celiac disease, gluten immunogenic peptides (GIP), gluten-free diet (GFD) follow-up, POCT gluten contamination, gluten-free products

1. Introduction

Celiac disease (CD), also known as gluten-sensitive enteropathy or celiac sprue, is a common immune-mediated inflammatory disease that primarily affects the small intestine caused by an autoimmune response to dietary gluten and related proteins in genetically predisposed individuals, with the human leukocyte antigen, HLA-DQ2, and/or HLA-DQ8 haplotypes. It is estimated that approximately 0.5 to 2 percent of the population around the world is affected by this condition [1–5].

Hence, pathogenesis of CD depends on genetic and environmental factors. The main environmental factor is the gluten intake [6]. Digestion of gluten in the gastro-intestinal tract generates immunoactive peptides, of which the 33-mer of alfa-gliadin (p57–68) has become a reference for its resistant to digestion and specific activity [7]. For simplification of the huge variability of peptides that are generated, the gluten digested fractions that could stimulate T cell in most celiac patients, they are referred as gluten immunogenic peptides (GIP) [7–9].

GIP that are encountered in the CD patients gut lumen, cross to the lamina propria using either the transcellular or paracellular path, leading to the activation of both adaptive and innate immune responses. This finally results in a structural change in the small intestinal mucosa, intraepithelial lymphocyte infiltration and in a defective digestion and malabsorption of nutrients, amongst others [6, 10].

CD clinical manifestations are highly variable, as it could range from the classical gastrointestinal symptoms (e.g., malabsorption, diarrhea, steatorrhea, weight loss, bloating, flatulence, abdominal pain), to extraintestinal symptoms (e.g., dermatitis herpetiformis, arthritis, neurological symptoms, anemia, osteopenia, osteoporosis, tooth enamel defects, aphthous stomatitis, hypertransaminasemia) or with no symptoms at all [1, 6, 11]. Moreover, in the worst cases, when the disease remains undetected or not treated properly, it is associated with an increased risk of bone fracture or intestinal lymphoma [10, 12].

Currently, the unique available treatment for CD is to adhere to a strict lifelong GFD. Once the dietary treatment is established, CD associated symptoms, and risks of long-term complications, decrease, as the histology of the small bowel architecture is restored. Different studies have shown that the 95% of the children achieved a complete mucosal healing after two years of a GDF follow-up, whereas in adults a 34% and 66% accomplished duodenal mucosal recovery after two and five years, respectively [12, 13].

2. Is a complete removal of gluten from the diet achievable?

GFD should be mainly based on natural foods without gluten: fruits, vegetables, legumes, gluten-free pseudocereals (rice, corn, millet, sorghum, buckwheat, amaranth and quinoa), tubers, meat, fish, nuts and dairy products. This food selection can be supplemented with certified gluten-free products, whose purpose is to replace foods traditionally made with gluten, such as bread, pasta, pastries, etc. [14, 15].

Despite the GFD efficacy, a significant number of CD patients does not report a good adherence to the treatment [6]. Several studies based on serological tests, dietetic questionnaires and GIP detection in stool and urine, revealed that up to 45% of the children, 64% of the teenagers and 69% of adults commit diet transgressions whilst following the GFD [13, 16]. It has been estimated that the mean exposure to gluten in many patients may exceed 100 mg/day, which may be sufficient to produce persistent symptoms, enteropathy, and long-term complications [17, 18].

Effectively, going on a strict GFD is an arduous task, unimaginable elements such as lipsticks or plasticine also might be composed of gluten. The adherence to GF-life implies on the one hand, a deep understanding of the condition and gluten ubiquity by the patients and their closest social circles. On the other hand, GFD implicates sensory, nutritional, motivational, social, and economic difficulties [6, 19–21].

Naturally, gluten immunoactive peptides can be mainly found in wheat, rye and barley, which are widely used to make food products such as bread, beer, pasta, cakes, pastries and biscuits. Despite the low nutritional and biological value of this protein mixtures, it is, after sugar, the most used additive in industry [22, 23]. Its multiple properties, thermostability, the fact that it can act as a binding and extending agent, it can hold moisture and improve flavors and textures (it can be used as thickener, emulsifier, or gelling agent) make of it an excellent additive. Thus, less obvious gluten sources include processed foods (e.g., snacks or reconstituted meat and seafood), medications and cosmetic products [23]. Equally important is to be aware of cross-contaminations which can easily occur by contacting other foods that contain gluten or by using the same utensils to cook or manipulate one and the other without sanitizing them properly [14].

In sensorial and nutritional terms, GF food is not preferred versus their gluten containing versions. Industry efforts to make tastier and with nicer textures make those products higher in carbohydrates and lipids, mainly saturated fat, thus resulting in high-calorie foods which give high glycaemic index (GIP) [24, 25]. Moreover, because of the development of new formulas, a shorter shelf-life, the need of special packaging due to a higher microbial and fungal contamination risk, cleanings for GF manufacturing lines and accreditations for labelling as GF food amongst others, makes this food 200–500% more expensive than their gluten-containing counterparts [19, 24]. What for instance for a Spanish coeliac citizen translates into an increasement of 1000€ in its shopping card per year [26]. Some countries as Italy, Canada or the USA offer a gluten-free tax or subsidies deduction for those who are on a GFD for proven medical reasons [27].

CD is also associated with increased risk of suffering some psychiatric conditions as depression, anxiety, eating disorders, autistic spectrum disorder (ASD) and attention deficit hyperactivity disorder (ADHD). It is argued that some of them are developed by a specific biological mechanism by a "gut-brain" relationship, and others are developed indirectly for the social and motivational implications involved [28]. After starting the GFD, as CD related symptoms improve, the incidence of anxiety and depression in celiac patients decreases. However, after certain period, the psychological conditions increase again, probably due to the difficulties to match the professional and social life with the requirements of the diet. Isolation, shame, fear of becoming contaminated by gluten and worries about being a bother are common amongst CD patients [29].

From all the above, the achieved adherence is strongly associated with cognitive, emotional, and socio-cultural issues, membership of an advocacy group and regular dietetic follow-up [20]. Therefore, it is important that the coeliac has psychological, nutritional, caregivers and social support and on hand tools to adapt and continue with excellent adherence to the gluten-free diet.

3. How much gluten is harmful in celiac disease without significant clinical consequences?

The difficulty of absolute adhesion to the GFD makes patients to frequently ask doctors how much gluten they may tolerate.

Over the last years several studies have tried to answer to this very demanded question. Although the responses obtained differ, probably because methodology differences amongst studies, some studies support that small daily amounts of <50 mg could be tolerated by most celiac patients. However, for some of the patients amounts as little as 10 mg per day could lead to an immunological and histological response [30–32].

Those studies mentioned above were done involving a gluten challenge, meaning a certain amount of gluten was administered daily. The frequency to which those voluntary and/or involuntary gluten exposures occurs may be even more relevant to cause persistent histological damage than occasional high gluten intake [31, 33].

There is unfortunately not a simple answer to the question of this section that can be given to all patients. Ultimately, different gluten intake patterns may lead to negative impact on celiac patients. Studying patients on a case-by-case basis could be a very time-consuming trial and inaccurate. To facilitate this task, both sides, healthcare providers and patients, should be provided with the correct tools and appropriate monitoring methodology to find the tolerable threshold for each patient. Otherwise, a single response would be offered: following GFD as strict as possible.

4. Current tools and strategies to measure the adherence to the GFD

In case of children and teenagers, ESPGHAN guidelines recommend follow-up visits after CD diagnosis. The first one should be programmed 3-–6 months after. Then, subsequent visits should be taken every 6 months until normalization of TGA levels, and every 12–24 months thereafter, unless there are concerns, complications or symptoms do persist and a sooner review is needed [3]. Likewise, there are similar universal agreement for adults [1, 2, 4, 5].

The aim of this monitorization is to evaluate the adherence to the treatment (GFD) and to detect any complication, which can be done either directly asking for the diet followed or fecal/urine GIP determinations, or indirectly, observing the clinical evolution from diagnosis (symptoms persistence, nutritional status and new clinic manifestations or associated complications) [16, 34, 35]. For this purpose, the following tools are used in clinical practice:

4.1 Clinical assessment

Once the GFD has been established, it is analyzed if symptoms and risk of complications have decreased, and quality of life is enhanced [2]. Despite a decrease in symptoms is associated with a response to the GFD, it has some weak points. On the one hand, several studies have stated that is an unreliable marker regarding recovery from intestinal atrophy [32, 36–39]. On the other hand, there are patients who are asymptomatic or express insignificant symptomatology, for whom the clinical assessment cannot be used as treatment monitoring indicator [36].

Additionally, other causes may motivate GI symptoms that could be easily confused with CD symptoms [37]. Therefore, clinical symptoms should not be considered as reliable method to evaluate the adherence to the GFD.

4.2 Dietetic review

Regular or periodical visits to an experienced dietitian in CD are recommended by different world-known guides [5, 35]. Relying on professional guidance is considered as key driver to accomplish the GFD. In order to evaluate the compliance grade, professionals are informed from patients' self-reports, for which the Standardized Dietician Evaluation [SDE] is commonly used, and on CD specialized dietetic questionnaires [16], such as, the Celiac Dietary Adherence Test [CDAT] or the Biagi Score [38, 40, 41].

Despite they have been advocated for being cost-effective and not invasive, they show some limitations. Firstly, questionnaires need to be translated and validated in all languages and cultures and do not register gluten real consumption. Secondly, self-reports are imprecise and subjective, as they depend on the patient's knowledge about the GFD and its fear to be judged [11, 42]. All these limitations resulted in the poor sensitivity of the dietary questionnaires to predict either villus atrophy or poor adherence in adult patients [39, 43].

Owing to those limitations, scientific research advocates more for the use of these tools to provide education for the avoidance of future inadvertent gluten exposures [36].

4.3 Endoscopy with duodenal biopsies

Duodenal biopsies provided by expert personnel or image analysis by advance technologies give a direct idea of the state of the GI mucosa. Either Marsh-Oberhuber classification or changes in villous height: crypt depth ratio (Vh:Cd) are used for its evaluation [44].

Despite current guidelines suggest follow-up biopsies every 1–2 years when symptoms persist, its use is frequently debated [1, 5, 35, 45]. On the one hand, endoscopies are invasive, expensive and need of experienced professionals to be done and interpreted and/or alternatively, specialized equipment to control biopsies and Vh:Cd determinations. On the other hand, despite an apparent strict compliance with GFD, mucosal damage could persist for years in certain adults [36, 39]. Therefore, the use of endoscopy in the follow-up tends to be more reduced.

4.4 Antibody-type serological biomarkers

Anti-gliadin antibody (anti-AGA), anti-endomysial antibody (anti-EMA), anti-tissue transglutaminase (anti-tTG)- TG2, TG6, TG3 and anti-deamidated gliadin peptide (anti-DGP), are the specific serologic antibody biomarkers in CD [46, 47].

Whereas their presence and their level above certain concentrations (e.g., anti-TG2 $\geq$ 10 times above the upper limit of baseline level), are very useful in the diagnosis of CD with a high sensitivity and specificity, they are not convenient biomarkers to check during the follow-up because of the low sensitivity [3, 39, 43]. Negative results are achieved with a reduction of gluten consumption, but frequent low quantities of gluten can also reduce the antibody level. Most of the individuals who do not portray a strict adherence to the GFD but do reduce the level of gluten consumption could also lead to a normalization of serology, without achieving a mucosal healing [1, 39, 47].

Other reasons that need also to bear in mind when using the serological biomarkers in the follow-up are:

- Cross-reaction with antibodies of enteric infections, other autoimmune diseases or chronic conditions may happen leading to false positive results [45].

- Once the GFD is prescribed, it usually takes $\geq$6–24 months to negativize. Some of them never reach full normalization of the serology. The timing of normalization can significantly vary amongst individuals [35].

- Patients with general or specific immunodeficiencies (in IgA or IgG) would lead to false negative results [45].

4.5 Novel biomarkers

The methods mentioned above have some weaknesses regarding GFD follow-up. Therefore, a general accepted tool for the follow-up of CD is still pending to be available. The following biomarkers are providing new information and advantages over the traditional tools [46, 48]:

4.5.1 Interleukin-2 (IL-2)

To be diagnosed with CD through conventional strategies it is mandatory that the patients are ingesting enough gluten in their diet [1, 3]. However, thanks to the increase in popular awareness of celiac disease and other gluten or wheat related conditions, many of the people who suspect that gluten is causing damage to them, reduce or suppress gluten in the diet before they are diagnosed. Consequently, the people on GFD are asked to go through a gluten challenge, which consists of long gluten exposure periods, for example, children are asked for three-months gluten challenge, to provoke intestinal damage and increasement of CD specific antibodies [1, 3]. Due to physical discomfort caused by this challenge in many people, it raises a lot of rejection and/or abandonment. Therefore, interest in new diagnostic techniques for the population on GFD is growing [48, 49].

Despite those new CD diagnosing techniques still need significant daily gluten consumption, those are based on bigger intakes in shorter periods of time, counted in days. These provocations are not centred in altering the gastrointestinal mucosal state or CD specific antibodies by itself, but the initiation of an unleashing of messengers, molecules, cells of the innate and adaptive immunity that can serve as biomarkers in the diagnosis of CD in people with GFD [48, 49].

Serum IL-2 is one of the most consistently upregulated cytokines in celiac patients, peaking 4 hours after consumption of gluten containing foods and becoming undetectable for most of the patients by 6 days after initial gluten exposure. Likewise, it is correlated with timing and severity of symptoms [35, 46, 50].

However, interleukins are a type of cytokine, molecules released by the immune system that are used for signaling amongst cells, not only in CD but many other conditions. T CD4+ and CD8+ activated cells are the mayor sources of IL-2. IL-2 regulates the activities of white blood cells responsible for immunity [51]. Therefore, the use of IL-2 in the follow-up by its own it is controversial, it would be more clarifying to look at a panel of biomarkers that are up- or down-regulated during gluten exposure in celiac patients.

4.5.2 Gluten-specific CD4 T cells

Gluten-specific CD4 T cells which have a central role on CD pathogenesis, are released into the blood 6 days after the start of a three-day gluten challenge. Those gluten-specific T cells can be detected by gIFN ELISpot, IP-10 ELISA or visualized by flow cytometry [48].

4.5.3 Urinary and fecal gluten immunogenic peptides

GIPs generated after glutens gastrointestinal partial hydrolysis, contain sequences that are immunoactive in CD patients. The presence in stools or urine of gluten peptides is a direct proof of previous gluten consumption. Those GIP can be detected by immunomethods developed from food analytical products,

GIP can be detected either in urine and stool after 2–15 hours and 12–120 hours of gluten intakes, respectively, by using immunoassays in LFIA and ELISA platforms. As low as 50 mg gluten intakes could be detected [52, 53]. The fact that GIPs gave an objective precise approach for determining voluntary or involuntary gluten consumption has made of them to be increasingly used in clinical trials of non-dietary therapies of CD, and studies with healthy and celiac children and adults [39, 43, 54–57]. Despite the undeniable direct association and effectiveness of the novel biomarkers to predict adherence to GFD, they are still not broadly implemented in the field.

4.5.4 Comparison of the current tools for GFD follow-up

The table showed below (**Table 1**) summarizes the most used current tools for GFD follow-up, presenting the advantages and disadvantages of each technique.

The curation of celiac patient could be considered when it achieves a complete mucosal healing, however, the risk of gluten exposure to deteriorate unremittingly the intestinal mucosa is always a threat. This complete healing process can only be accomplished by a full adherence to a GFD. The timing that would take for a complete recovery could vary patient to patient.

GFD assessment tool	Advantages	Disadvantages
Clinical assessment	1. Cheap. 2. Not invasive.	1. It cannot be used with asymptomatic patients, which may represent about two thirds of the CD population. 2. The symptoms caused must be differentiated from the ones that might have other origins. 3. Unreliable regarding recovery from intestinal atrophy.
Dietetic review	1. No requirement of instrumentation. 2. Not invasive. 3. Availability of standardized questionnaires.	1. Must be translated and validated in all languages and cultures. 2. Time consuming 3. Imprecise and subjective, as they are subject to the responses of each patient 4. Poor sensitivity to predict either villus atrophy and adherence
Endoscopy with duodenal biopsies	1. Determination of the gluten intake consequences through checking GI mucosal state.	1. Expensive 2. Invasive 3. Need either of experienced professionals or form specialized equipment 4. The reversibility of the damage can vary in time from patient to patient
Antibody type serological biomarkers	1. Cost effective. 2. Positive results might indicate continuous exposure to normal gluten containing diets.	1. Semi-invasive 2. Negative values in most treated patients with gluten exposure. Low sensitivity. 3. Cannot be used with immunocompromised patients 4. False positives might be obtained due to crossreactions with other antibodies 5. The timing of normalization can significantly vary amongst individuals 6. There is no linear correlation between serology values and recovery of the intestinal mucosa

GFD assessment tool	Advantages	Disadvantages
Interleukin-2	Low evidence for the utility in the follow-up.	
Gluten-specific CD4 T cells		1. Expensive instrument. 2. Required highly skilled technicians.
Gluten immunogenic peptides	1. Cost effective 2. Non-invasive. 3. Direct indicator that a gluten intake has been committed. 4. May help to identify the source of gluten exposure. 5. May estimate the amount of gluten consumption	1. Window of detection per sample is limited to hoursdays. 2. May require multiple samples (at least two) to increase accuracy and reliability.

Table 1.
Advantages and disadvantages of the existing current tools for GFD adherence assessment.

5. Can GIP determinations be the "gold standard" for exploring adherence?

In contrast to the rest of the presented methods, GIPs determination is the only tool that directly evidences the gluten intake whilst the rest of them try to determine the consequences.

5.1 What are the peptides included in the term?

Any gluten peptide that has immunoactivity with CD patients' T cells can be considered a GIP [58].

Since GIP have been detected in feces and urine, they probably could be located along the gastrointestinal tract and/or blood [59].

GIP present in stool and urine are derived from the digestion process. When gluten is ingested, it is partially digested to different size oligopeptides by digestive enzymes [60]. However, there are certain sequences that could be resistant to gastrointestinal digestion by the hydrolytic enzymes from human, such as, the immunodominant 33-mer alpha gliadin peptide, which has demonstrated to be resistant to gastric, pancreatic and intestinal brush-border membrane proteases [7]. Gluten is a protein rich in proline (P) and glutamine (Q) amino acids, what gives it its hydrophobic quality and at the same time it makes certain of those P and Q rich sequences hard to digest. Some of those indigestible sequences have the capacity of triggering an immune response in CD patients [60, 61].

During the last decades, considerable efforts have been made to map coeliac immunogenic motifs, a work that from time to time, is updated to add newly found gluten immunogenic sequences to the hundreds that have already been described as such [62]. Some immunogenic gluten epitopes may be tolerated at different level depending on the CD patient, as each person may have a different sensitivity towards the different epitopes [30, 32]. It has been demonstrated T cells have more affinity by the peptides presented by the HLA-DQ2 complexes than the ones presented by HLA-DQ8 ones. Therefore, the immune system response between individuals who have one or the other molecule would also be different [63]. However, it must be stated that not all gluten peptides are involved in the development of CD, as some may not contain immunogenic sequences. The immunogenicity of each GIP for T cell activation could be variable depending on the specificity and repetitions of immunogenic T cell epitopes [63, 64]. This amount can easily vary depending on the peptide's gluten source. Hence, the 33-mer of the alpha-2-gladin is recognized for being the most immunodominant gluten peptide and used to be the referent GIP in analytical determinations. It contains three overlapping T-cell epitopes, namely PFPQPQLPY (DQ2.5-glia-α1a, one copy), PYPQPQLPY (DQ2.5-glia-α1b, two copies) and PQPQLPYPQ (DQ2.5-glia-α2, three copies) [61]. The deamidation of certain glutamine residues by the TG2 enhances the immunogenicity. TG2 has preference for QxP sites, where x, can be any amino acid [65].

5.2 Methods to determine GIP in human specimen

GIP have been detected in stool by ELISA and LFIA [43]. LC–MS, SPR, ELISA and LFIA [43, 59, 66, 67] have shown to determine urine GIP. Each method shows a different level of sensitivity and simplicity of execution.

The described methods for SPR, ELISA and LFIA to detect GIP in human stool and urine are immunoassays based on the G12 and/or A1 antibodies.

The study made by Palanski *et al.*, [59] with LC–MS described for the first time the kind of gluten derived peptides that could be found in urine after gluten intake. The smallest peptide had 1,33 KDa and the largest was 4,28 KDa, for non-CD people after the intake of 18 g of gluten. 10/16 of these peptides showed at least 1 epitope for A1, 6/10 for G12 and 6/16 for both (**Table 2**). GIPs in stool have not been described so far.

Molecular size (KDa)	Sequence	Nº of epitopes for G12	Nº of epitopes for A1	Nº of volunteers that was encountered
4.28	SQQPEQTISQ**QPQQPFP**QQPH**QPQQPY**PQQQPYGSSL	2	1	6/8
3.46	PQQPPFSQQQQQQQQQQPPFSQQQQPVL	0	0	3/8
3.41	PyrQQQQPPFSQQPPISQQQQPPFSQQQQPQF	0	0	1/8
3.33	TQ**QPQQPFP**QQ**PQQPFP**QTQ**QPQQPFP**Q	3	2	3/8
3.15	FL**QPQQPFP**QQ**PQQPY**PQ**QPQQPF**PQ	3	1	1/8
3.10	TQ**QPQQPFP**QQ**PQQPFP**QQ**PQQPFP**Q	3	2	3/8
2.76	LGQQQPFPP**QQPYPQP**QPFPSQQP	0	1	5/8
2.51	SQ**QPQQPFP**QQPH**QPQQPY**PQ	2	1	5/8
2.35	P[I/L]**QPQQPFP**QQ**PQQPFP**QPQc	2	2	2/8
2.35	PyrQTFPHQPQQQVPQPQQPQQP	0	0	5/8
2.29	GQQQPFPPQQPYPQPQPFPS	0	1	8/8
2.21	GQQQPFPPQQPYPQPQPFP	0	1	7/8
1.89	QPFPPQQPYPQPQPFP	0	1	2/8
1.46	SCHVMQQQCCQ	0	0	5/8
1.39	CHVMQQQCCQd	0	0	1/8
1.33	SCHVMQQQCC	0	0	6/8

Table 2.
Modified from Palanski et al., *[59]. Gluten derived peptide sequences found in urine that show epitopes for G12, in bold and for A1 in red.*

Both A1 and G12 antibodies do not only detect gluten derived epitopes present in the α-gliadin 33-mer, but detect most immunogenic peptides [61, 68]. Furthermore, the G12 monoclonal antibody, has shown to capture most of the immunoactivity of digested gluten from different sources with an immunoaffinity resin [58, 68, 69],

Products for measuring GIP in feces and urine are currently on the market, adapted for both professional and domestic use [43]. Those ones for home use are based on the LFIA, whose mechanism of use and interpretation of the results are simple and already well known by the general population due to the familiarity of this type of test during the COVID-19 pandemic. Kits for professional use were designed in ELISA and LFIA formats, methods routinely used in clinical laboratories with the potential to provide quantitative data of GIP concentration. Facilitating user-adapted detection, allows GIP to be used as a biomarker of GFD adherence by both, professionals who perform the patient's follow-up and by the patient itself. In this way, they can detect failures and improve adherence to their treatment. Those kits are commercialized by the names of GlutenDetect Urine and Stool, LFIA for domestic use, iVYCHECK GIP Stool and iVYCHECK GIP Urine, LFIA for professional use and iVYLISA GIP Stool, ELISA for professional use.

The LFIA test for detecting GIP in urine has a LLoQ of 2.5 ng GIP/mL, for stool in stool is 0.3 μg GIP/g feces, where the LLoQ was established as the rate in which the 95% of the samples to that concentration get a positive result, using as a measurand the 33-mer (**Figure 1**). Those LFIA are semiqualitative tests, generally providing a binary result "positive" or "negative" that can be easily interpreted. However, they have been also conveniently used for semi-quantitative determination with a lateral flow reader.

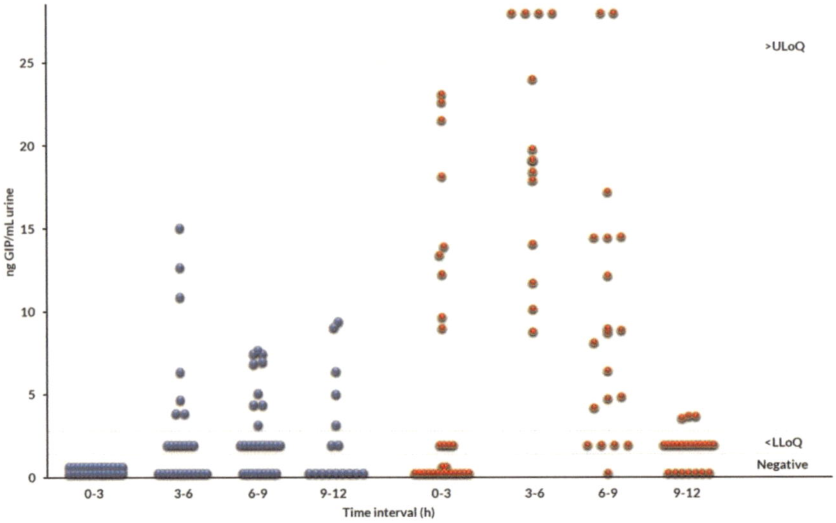

Figure 1.
Urinations collected after 2 g of encapsuled [52] and 8 g of free gluten intake, represented with blue and red spots respectively, during a 12 hours' time lapse, presented in 3 hours intervals (0–3 h, 3–6 h, 6–9 h and 9–12 h) for GIP detection and quantification. The urinations come from 21 healthy individuals for 2 g intake and from 15 healthy individuals for 8 g intake. For the dynamic range allowed, there were some urines that were positive de visu *but undetectable for the reader, those urines are the ones on the <LLoQ range; the ones on the >ULoQ are the ones detectable by the reader but whose concentration was undistinguishable. The negative urines are given the concentration below 2 ng GIP/mL.*

The ELISA test for detecting GIP in stool has a LLoQ of 0,3 μg α-gliadin 33mer/g feces. The ELISA test is a semi-quantitative method. Therefore, it allows to differentiate those stools for their GIP content within a dynamic range.

The reproducibility, repeatability and the diagnostic features of those tests are summarized in the table below (**Table 3**):

	iVYCHECK GIP Urine	iVYCHECK GIP Stool	iVYLISA GIP Stool
Diagnostic sensitivity *	90.18% (95%IC: 84.22–96.14%)	94.60% (95%IC: 86.00–100%)	97.10% (95%IC: 90.20–100%)
Diagnostic specificity *	98.28% (95%IC: 95.48–100%)	100% (95%IC: 98.80–100%)	83.30% (95%IC: 63.30–100%)
Positive predictive value *	98.06% (95%IC: 94.91–100%)	100% (95%IC: 98.60–100%)	91.90% (95%IC: 81.80–100%)
Negative predictive value *	91.20% (95%IC: 85.83–96.57%)	95.20% (95%IC: 87.60–100%)	93.75% (95%IC: 78.80–100%)
Reproducibility	97.00% (95%IC: 95.00–98.00%)	98.00% (95%IC: 96.00–99.00%)	CV ≤ 22%
Repeatability	98.00% (95%IC: 94.00–100%)	98.00% (95%IC: 94.00–100%)	CV ≤ 17%

**Associated with people without restrictions on gluten consumption in the diet. Intake not controlled.*

Table 3.
Features of the urine and stool GIP detecting kits in the market for professional use.

5.3 How [when] to collect samples for GIP determinations

The timing for the sampling is an important issue to maximize outcomes. The understanding of the GIP excretion dynamics helps us to select the most convenient time window in which this involuntary ingestion/transgression occurred [52, 53, 70] and even models have been made to estimate the relative amount of this transgression [17].

The studies by Coto *et al.*, [52, 53] with healthy volunteers, and Burger *et al.*, with celiac patients [70] had allowed us to know some key issues about the dynamics of GIP excretion (related to single-dose intakes of gluten) in feces and urine (**Table 4**):

	Stool		Urine
	LFIA	ELISA	LFIA
Minimum gluten intake amount that has been detected (single dose)	50 mg	50 mg	50 mg
Excretion window for 50 mg	12–84 h	0–84 h	3–12 h
Excretion window for 2 g	0–132 h	12–204 h	1–15 h
Peak of GIP (time after gluten intake)	24–48 h	24–48 h	6–9 h

Table 4.
Summary of the performance of GIP detecting test according to GIP excretion dynamics.

In feces, GIP excretion is delayed for at least 1 day and wash out in 2–7 days, whilst in urine the excretion peak occurs earlier, and it is narrower than for stool. In feces, as expected, a higher consumption of gluten was correlated to a higher concentration of

GIP in the sample, and to a longer detection period after single gluten intake. In urine the excretion of gluten over time behaves in a similar way regardless of the consumption, with a higher variability on the GIP concentration than in feces (**Figure 1**) [39, 52, 53].

Regarding those differences, it could be assumed that feces are presented as a more convenient sample for a dietary practice evaluation, whereas urine would facilitate the identification of a punctual transgression and would require multiple samples to assess routine diet. As a counterpoint, it is convenient to bear in mind that patients and laboratory professionals are often reluctant to collect and use stool samples, and that for the optimal use of urine, the time relationship between the expected gluten exposure and sample collection must be considered.

In addition, visualizing these generalized behaviors, recommendation of use based on time and the amount of gluten ingested/GIP detected have been generated to help for a better understanding and interpretation of the results obtained [52, 53].

Likewise, it is necessary to understand that each individual works as a different bioreactor and that, although certain behavior patterns can be established, not everyone will do it in the same way. However, there will be certain factors that can be controlled to reduce this inter-individual variability, such as fluid intake or time of the day to collect the samples [52].

6. What would be a practical strategy for assessing adherence by using GIP determinations?

The presence of GIP, either in a urine or stool sample, is a direct indicative that a gluten intake has been committed in the previous hours or days to the sample collection, respectively [52, 53, 70].

The frequency (daily or occasional), the amount of immunoactive gluten to which a celiac is exposed, and the individual sensitivity to GIP have a direct impact on the recovery of the gastrointestinal mucosa.

The dynamic of GIP excretion, average harmful gluten exposure (0.1–0.5 g daily gluten intake for celiac population), distribution of daily meals, analytical sensitivity of the immunoassays, individual variability in metabolisms and habits, studies of correlation of GIP multitesting results with villus atrophy, practical issues and statistical analysis of the results, have been considered to propose protocols of the assessment GFD adherence tests and interpretation of the results with the two kind of samples [30, 33, 52, 53, 57].

Urine GIP: Determination of the presence/absence of GIP in three different urine samples a week, collected with an interval of two days, and at least one of the three having been collected on a weekend. The work led by Ruiz-Carnicer *et al.*, where 77 celiac patients who had been on at least a two-year GFD participated, showed that urine tests had a diagnostic sensitivity of 94.4% regarding villous atrophy when the three urine samples collected during the same week had GIP presence. Two out of three of those urines were collected at the weekend, Saturday, and Sunday, and the third one on the day of the medical visit. With this protocol, negative predictive values for intestinal mucosa recovery of 3/3 negative urine GIP reached 97% in this study [39, 52].

Fecal GIP: Determinations of GIP presence/absence in two different stool samples a week, collected with an interval of three to four days, and at least one being representative of the consumptions during the weekend [70–73].

Thus, the studies carried out have made it possible to establish different degrees of adherence to treatment according to the number of samples in which GIP have been found, making three classifications: "excellent adherent," "good adherent" or "poor adherent" [39].

ELISA tests allowed to establish a GIP concentration value for the stool samples, and it has been stipulated that the finding of values higher than 0.6 μg GIP/g feces point to poor adherents which may increase risk of villus atrophy [71, 72].

If it is understood that humans are animals of habits and customs, the determination of GIP in three urines or two stools in the same week, is a practical and objective procedure to perform assessment of the celiac patient's adherence to the treatment. GIP detection allows to distinguish the degree of compliance of the patient to the prescribed diet, and predict its probability to cure or remission, probably even before long-term damage. Furthermore, several studies have showed that the repeated presence of GIP correlated higher with the duodenal mucosal damage than the traditional tools for monitoring adherence to the GFD such as serology, symptomatology, or dietary questionnaires [39].

In conclusion, GIP determinations, following a clinical validated protocol, appear to be a cost-effective, non-invasive, objective and straight forward strategy to assess GFD adherence. In addition, it may allow to predict with some accuracy when the gluten ingestion has been committed, which may enable to identify the source of gluten contamination. That information would serve to prevent future repetition of gluten exposure, improving the chances for a full GFD adherence and complete intestinal mucosa recovery. The GIP presence in human excretions is the direct evidence that the cause of the toxicity in CD, the gluten peptides, has been circulating in the patient body. At this point, does it makes sense to investigate alternative endpoints to proof deficiencies in the dietary treatment of the celiac disease?

Acknowledgements

Supported by Ministerio de Ciencia e Innovación, No. DI-17-09627.
Grant funded by CTA (22/1075) and CDTI (IDI-20220676).
Grant DI-17-09627 funded by MCIN/AEI/10.13039/501100011033.

Conflict of interest

Ángel Cebolla is the founder and current CEO of Biomedal S.L., and it is the co-inventor of the patent "Detecting gluten peptides in human fluids" No. WO/2016/005643.

Irati Mendia is employee at Biomedal S.L.

Appendices and Nomenclature

ADHD	attention deficit hyperactivity disorder
ASD	autistic spectrum disorder
anti-AGA	Anti-gliadin antibody
anti-EMA	anti-endomysial antibody
anti-tTG	anti-tissue transglutaminase

CDAT	Celiac Dietary Adherence Test
CD	Celiac Disease
ELISA	Enzyme linked immunosorbent assay
ESPGHAN	The European Society for Pediatric Gastroenterology Hepatology and Nutrition
GF	Gluten Free
GFD	Gluten Free Diet
GI	Gastrointestinal
GIP	Gluten Immunogenic Peptides
IL-2	Interleukin-2
LFIA	Lateral flow immunoassay
LC-MS	Liquid chromatography–mass spectrometry
LLoQ	Lower limit of quantification
ULoQ	Upper limit of quantification
POCT	Point-of-care testing
SPR	Surface plasmon resonance
TG2	anti-tissue transglutaminase type 2
Vh:Cd	Villous height: crypt depth ratio

Author details

Irati Mendia Azkoaga[1*] and Ángel Cebolla[2]

1 Biomedal SL, University of Seville, Seville, Spain

2 Biomedal SL, Seville, Spain

*Address all correspondence to: irati.mendia@biomedal.com

References

[1] Rubio-Tapia A, Hill ID, Kelly CP, Calderwood AH, Murray JA. ACG clinical guidelines: Diagnosis and management of celiac disease. The American Journal of Gastroenterology. 2013;**108**(5):656-676

[2] Al-Toma A, Volta U, Auricchio R, Castillejo G, Sanders DS, Cellier C, et al. European Society for the Study of coeliac disease (ESsCD) guideline for coeliac disease and other gluten-related disorders. United European Gastroenterology Journal. 2019;**7**(5): 583-613

[3] Mearin ML, Agardh D, Antunes H, Al-Toma A, Auricchio R, Castillejo G, et al. ESPGHAN position paper on management and follow-up of children and adolescents with celiac disease. Journal of Pediatric Gastroenterology and Nutrition. 2022;**75**(3):369-386

[4] Husby S, Murray JA, Katzka DA. AGA clinical practice update on diagnosis and monitoring of celiac disease: Changing utility of serology and histologic measures: Expert review. Gastroenterology. 2019;**156**(4):885-889

[5] Raiteri A, Granito A, Giamperoli A, Catenaro T, Negrini G, Tovoli F. Current guidelines for the management of celiac disease: A systematic review with comparative analysis. World Journal of Gastroenterology. 2022;**28**(1): 154-175

[6] Lindfors K, Ciacci C, Kurppa K, Lundin KEA, Makharia GK, Mearin ML, et al. Coeliac disease. Nature Reviews Disease Primers. 2019;**5**(1):3

[7] Shan L, Molberg Ø, Parrot I, et al. Structural basis for gluten intolerance in celiac sprue. Science. 2002;**297**(5590): 2275-2279

[8] Sollid LM, Qiao S-W, Anderson RP, Gianfrani C, Koning F. Nomenclature and listing of celiac disease relevant gluten T-cell epitopes restricted by HLA-DQ molecules. Immunogenetics. 2012; **64**(6):455-460

[9] Fleckenstein B, Molberg Ø, Qiao SW, Schmid DG, Von Mülbe F. Der, Elgstøen K, et al. gliadin T cell epitope selection by tissue transglutaminase in celiac disease. Role of enzyme specificity and pH influence on the transamidation versus deamidation reactions. The Journal of Biological Chemistry. 2002; **277**(37):34109-34116

[10] Tye-Din JA, Galipeau HJ, Agardh D. Celiac disease: A review of current concepts in pathogenesis, prevention, and novel therapies. Frontiers in Pediatrics. 2018;**6**:1-19

[11] Caio G, Volta U, Sapone A, Leffler DA, De Giorgio R, Catassi C, et al. Celiac disease: A comprehensive current review. BMC Medicine. 2019; **17**(1):142

[12] Rubio-Tapia A, Rahim MW, See JA, Lahr BD, Wu TT, Murray JA. Mucosal recovery and mortality in adults with celiac disease after treatment with a gluten-free diet. The American Journal of Gastroenterology. 2010;**105**(6):1412-1420

[13] Wahab PJ, Meijer JWR, Mulder CJJ. Histologic follow-up of people with celiac disease on a gluten-free diet: Slow and incomplete recovery. American Journal of Clinical Pathology. 2002; **118**(3):459-463

[14] Wieser H, Segura V, Ruiz-Carnicer Á, Sousa C, Comino I. Food safety and cross-contamination of gluten-free products: A narrative review. Nutrients. 2021;**13**(7):2244

[15] Rai S, Kaur A, Chopra CS. Gluten-free products for celiac susceptible people. Frontiers in Nutrition. 2018;**5** (December):1-23

[16] Wieser H, Ruiz-Carnicer Á, Segura V, Comino I, Sousa C. Challenges of monitoring the gluten-free diet adherence in the management and follow-up of patients with celiac disease. Nutrients. 2021;**13**(7):2274

[17] Syage JA, Kelly CP, Dickason MA, Ramirez AC, Leon F, Dominguez R, et al. Determination of gluten consumption in celiac disease patients on a gluten-free diet. The American Journal of Clinical Nutrition. 2018;**107**(2):201-207

[18] Comino I, Segura V, Ortigosa L, Espín B, Castillejo G, Garrote JA, et al. Prospective longitudinal study: Use of faecal gluten immunogenic peptides to monitor children diagnosed with coeliac disease during transition to a gluten-free diet. Alimentary Pharmacology & Therapeutics. 2019;**49**(12):1484-1492

[19] Mearns ES, Taylor A, Boulanger T, Craig KJ, Gerber M, Leffler DA, et al. Systematic literature review of the economic burden of celiac disease. PharmacoEconomics. 2019;**37**(1):45-61

[20] Hall NJ, Rubin G, Charnock A. Systematic review: Adherence to a gluten-free diet in adult patients with coeliac disease. Alimentary Pharmacology & Therapeutics. 2009; **30**(4):315-330

[21] Makharia GK, Singh P, Catassi C, et al. The global burden of coeliac disease: Opportunities and challenges. Nature Reviews. Gastroenterology & Hepatology. 2022;**19**(5):313-327. DOI: 10.1038/s41575-021-00552-z

[22] Consultation FAOE. Dietary protein quality evaluation in human nutrition. Report of an FAQ Expert Consultation. FAO Food and Nutrition Paper. 2013;**92**: 1-66

[23] Biesiekierski JR. What is gluten? Journal of Gastroenterology and Hepatology. 2017;**32**:78-81

[24] El Khoury D, Balfour-Ducharme S, Joye IJ. A review on the gluten-free diet: Technological and nutritional challenges. Nutrients. 2018;**10**(10):1-25

[25] Gobbetti M, Pontonio E, Filannino P, Rizzello CG, De Angelis M, Di Cagno R. How to improve the gluten-free diet: The state of the art from a food science perspective. Food Research International. 2018;**110**:22-32

[26] Federacion de Asociaciones de Celiacos de España. El gasto Anual Destinado a la Compra de Productos sin Gluten en 2022 ha Aumentado 86,97 €. [cited 2022 Nov 5]. Available from: https://celiacos.org/wp-content/uploads/2022/02/Ndp-Informe-de-precios-2022.pdf

[27] Economic Support for Coeliac People in the European Union | AOECS. [cited 2022 Nov 5]. Available from: https://www.aoecs.org/news/survey-on-economic-aid-for-coeliacs-in-europe/

[28] Clappison E, Hadjivassiliou M, Zis P. Psychiatric manifestations of coeliac disease, a systematic review and meta-analysis. Nutrients. 2020;**12**(1):10-15

[29] Sverker A, Hensing G, Hallert C. "Controlled by food" - lived experiences of coeliac disease. Journal of Human Nutrition and Dietetics. 2005;**18**(3): 171-180

[30] Catassi C, Fabiani E, Iacono G, D'Agate C, Francavilla R, Biagi F, et al. A prospective, double-blind, placebo-controlled trial to establish a safe gluten

threshold for patients with celiac disease. The American Journal of Clinical Nutrition. 2007;**85**(1):160-166

[31] Cohen IS, Day AS, Shaoul R. Gluten in celiac disease more or less? Rambam Maimonides Medical Journal. 2019; **10**(1):1-6

[32] Collin P, Thorell L, Kaukinen K, Mäki M. The safe threshold for gluten contamination in gluten-free products. Can trace amounts be accepted in the treatment of coeliac disease? Alimentary Pharmacology & Therapeutics. 2004; **19**(12):1277-1283

[33] Elli L, Bascuñán K, Di Lernia L, Bardella MT, Doneda L, Soldati L, et al. Safety of occasional ingestion of gluten in patients with celiac disease: A real-life study. BMC Medicine. 2020;**18**(1):1-8

[34] Elli L, Ferretti F, Orlando S, Vecchi M, Monguzzi E, Roncoroni L, et al. Management of celiac disease in daily clinical practice. European Journal of Internal Medicine. 2019;**61**:15-24

[35] Pinto-Sanchez MI, Bai JC. Toward new paradigms in the follow up of adult patients with celiac disease on a gluten-free diet. Frontiers in Nutrition. 2019;**6**: 153

[36] Sharkey LM, Corbett G, Currie E, Lee J, Sweeney N, Woodward JM. Optimising delivery of care in coeliac disease - comparison of the benefits of repeat biopsy and serological follow-up. Alimentary Pharmacology & Therapeutics. 2013;**38**(10):1278-1291

[37] Silvester JA, Graff LA, Rigaux L, Bernstein CN, Leffler DA, Kelly CP, et al. Symptoms of functional intestinal disorders are common in patients with celiac disease following transition to a gluten-free diet. Digestive Diseases and Sciences. 2017;**62**(9):2449-2454

[38] Leffler DA, Dennis M, Edwards George J, Jamma S, Cook EF, Schuppan D, et al. A validated disease-specific symptom index for adults with celiac disease. Clinical Gastroenterology and Hepatology. 2009;**7**(12):1328-1334.e3

[39] Ruiz-Carnicer A, Garzon-Benavides M, Fombuena B, Segura V, Garcia-Fernandez F, Sobrino-Rodriguez S, et al. Negative predictive value of the repeated absence of gluten immunogenic peptides in the urine of treated celiac patients in predicting mucosal healing: New proposals for follow-up in celiac disease. The American Journal of Clinical Nutrition. 2020;**112**(5):1240-1251

[40] Biagi F, Bianchi PI, Marchese A, Trotta L, Vattiato C, Balduzzi D, et al. A score that verifies adherence to a gluten-free diet: A cross-sectional, multicentre validation in real clinical life. The British Journal of Nutrition. 2012;**108**(10): 1884-1888

[41] Gładyś K, Dardzińska J, Guzek M, Adrych K, Małgorzewicz S. Celiac dietary adherence test and standardized dietician evaluation in assessment of adherence to a gluten-free diet in patients with celiac disease. Nutrients. 2020;**12**(8):1-10

[42] Silvester JA, Weiten D, Graff LA, Walker JR, Duerksen DR. Is it gluten-free? Relationship between self-reported gluten-free diet adherence and knowledge of gluten content of foods. Nutrition. 2016;**32**(7–8):777-783. DOI: 10.1016/j.nut.2016.01.021

[43] Comino I, Fernández-Bañares F, Esteve M, Ortigosa L, Castillejo G, Fambuena B, et al. Fecal gluten peptides reveal limitations of serological tests and food questionnaires for monitoring gluten-free diet in celiac disease patients. The American Journal of

Gastroenterology. 2016;**111**(10):1456-1465

[44] Adelman DC, Murray J, Wu T-T, Mäki M, Green PH, Kelly CP. Measuring change In small intestinal histology In patients with celiac disease. The American Journal of Gastroenterology. 2018;**113**(3):339-347

[45] Singh A, Pramanik A, Acharya P, Makharia GK. Non-invasive biomarkers for celiac disease. Journal of Clinical Medicine. 2019;**8**(6):1-17

[46] Castillo NE, Theethira TG, Leffler DA. The present and the future in the diagnosis and management of celiac disease. Gastroenterol Reports. 2015;**3**(1):3-11

[47] Vahedi K. Reliability of antitransglutaminase antibodies as predictors of gluten-free diet compliance in adult celiac disease. The American Journal of Gastroenterology. 2003;**98**(5):1079-1087

[48] Smithson G, Siegelman J, Oki T, Maxwell JR, Leffler DA. The evolving landscape of biomarkers in celiac disease: Leading the way to clinical development. Frontiers in Immunology. 2021;**12**:665-756

[49] Leonard MM, Silvester JA, Leffler D, et al. Evaluating responses to gluten challenge: A randomized, double-blind, 2-dose gluten challenge trial. Gastroenterology. 2021;**160**(3):720-733.e8. DOI: 10.1053/j.gastro.2020.10.040

[50] Tye-Din JA, Daveson AJM, Ee HC, Goel G, MacDougall J, Acaster S, et al. Elevated serum interleukin-2 after gluten correlates with symptoms and is a potential diagnostic biomarker for coeliac disease. Alimentary Pharmacology & Therapeutics. 2019;**50**(8):901-910

[51] Liao W, Lin JX, Leonard WJ. IL-2 family cytokines: New insights into the complex roles of IL-2 as a broad regulator of T helper cell differentiation. Current Opinion in Immunology. 2011;**23**(5):598-604

[52] Coto L, Sousa C, Cebolla A. Dynamics and considerations in the determination of the excretion of gluten immunogenic peptides in urine: Individual variability at low gluten intake. Nutrients. 2021;**13**(8):2624

[53] Coto L, Sousa C, Cebolla A. Individual variability in patterns and dynamics of fecal gluten immunogenic peptides excretion after low gluten intake. European Journal of Nutrition. 2022;**61**(4):2033-2049

[54] Silvester JA, Comino I, Kelly CP, Sousa C, Duerksen DR, DOGGIE BAG Study Group. Most patients with celiac disease on gluten-free diets consume measurable amounts of gluten. Gastroenterology. 2020;**158**(5):1497-1499.e1

[55] Murray JA, Syage JA, Wu TT, et al. Latiglutenase protects the mucosa and attenuates symptom severity in patients with celiac disease exposed to a gluten challenge. Gastroenterology. 2022;**163**(6):1510-1521

[56] Comino I, Real A, Vivas S, Síglez MÁ, Caminero A, Nistal E, et al. Monitoring of gluten-free diet compliance in celiac patients by assessment of gliadin 33-mer equivalent epitopes in faeces. The American Journal of Clinical Nutrition. 2012;**95**(3):670-677

[57] Coto L, Mendia I, Sousa C, Bai JC, Cebolla A. Determination of gluten immunogenic peptides for the management of the treatment adherence of celiac disease: A systematic review.

World Journal of Gastroenterology. 2021;**27**(37):6306-6321

[58] Murray JA, Syage JA, Wu TT, et al. Latiglutenase Protects the Mucosa and Attenuates Symptom Severity in Patients With Celiac Disease Exposed to a Gluten Challenge. Gastroenterology. 2022;**163**(6):1510-1521

[59] Palanski BA, Weng N, Zhang L, et al. An efficient urine peptidomics workflow identifies chemically defined dietary gluten peptides from patients with celiac disease. Nature Communications. 2022; **13**(1):88861

[60] Koning F. celiac disease: Quantity matters. Seminars in Immunopathology. 2012;**34**(4):541-549

[61] Schalk K, Lang C, Wieser H, Koehler P, Scherf KA. Quantitation of the immunodominant 33-mer peptide from α-gliadin in wheat flours by liquid chromatography tandem mass spectrometry. Scientific Reports. 2017; **7**(1):450-492

[62] Sollid LM, Tye-Din JA, Qiao SW, Anderson RP, Gianfrani C, Koning F. Update 2020: Nomenclature and listing of celiac disease–relevant gluten epitopes recognized by CD4+ T cells. Immunogenetics. 2020;**72**(1–2): 85-88

[63] Balakireva A, Zamyatnin A. Properties of gluten intolerance: Gluten structure, evolution, pathogenicity and detoxification capabilities. Nutrients. 2016;**8**(10):644

[64] Arentz-Hansen H, Mcadam SN, Molberg Ø, Fleckenstein B, KEA L, TJD J, et al. Celiac lesion T cells recognize epitopes that cluster in regions of gliadins rich in proline residues. Gastroenterology. 2002;**123**(3): 803-809

[65] Ciccocioppo R, Di Sabatino A, Corazza GR. The immune recognition of gluten in coeliac disease. Clinical and Experimental Immunology. 2005;**140** (3):408-416

[66] Peláez EC, Estevez M-C, Domínguez R, Sousa C, Cebolla A, Lechuga LM. A compact SPR biosensor device for the rapid and efficient monitoring of gluten-free diet directly in human urine. Analytical and Bioanalytical Chemistry. 2020;**412**(24): 6407-6417

[67] Soler M, Estevez M-C. Moreno M de L, Cebolla a, Lechuga LM. Label-free SPR detection of gluten peptides in urine for non-invasive celiac disease follow-up. Biosensors & Bioelectronics. 2016; **79**:158-164

[68] Morón B, Bethune MT, Comino I, Manyani H, Ferragud M, López MC, et al. Toward the assessment of food toxicity for celiac patients: Characterization of monoclonal antibodies to a main immunogenic gluten peptide. Zimmer J, editor. PLoS One. 2008;**3**(5):e2294

[69] Moreno ML, Muñoz-Suano A, López-Casado MÁ, Torres MI, Sousa C, Cebolla Á. Selective capture of most celiac immunogenic peptides from hydrolyzed gluten proteins. Food Chemistry. 2016;**205**:36-42

[70] Burger JPW, van Lochem EG, Roovers EA, Drenth JPH, Wahab PJ. Dose-escalating (50–500 mg) gluten administration leads to detectable gluten-immunogenic-peptides in urine of patients with coeliac disease which is unrelated to symptoms, a placebo controlled trial. Nutrients. 2022;**14**(9): 1771

[71] Stefanolo JP, Tálamo M, Dodds S, de la Paz TM, Costa AF, Moreno ML, et al.

Real-world gluten exposure in patients with celiac disease on gluten-free diets, determined from gliadin immunogenic peptides in urine and fecal samples. Clinical Gastroenterology and Hepatology. 2021;**19**(3):484-491

[72] Fernández-Bañares F, Beltrán B, Salas A, Comino I, Ballester-Clau R, Ferrer C, et al. Persistent villous atrophy in De novo adult patients with celiac disease and strict control of gluten-free diet adherence: A multicenter prospective study (CADER study). The American Journal of Gastroenterology. 2021;**116**(5):1036-1043

[73] Costa AF, Sugai E, Temprano M. de la P, Niveloni SI, Vázquez H, Moreno ML, et al. gluten immunogenic peptide excretion detects dietary transgressions in treated celiac disease patients. World Journal of Gastroenterology. 2019; **25**(11):1409-1420

Chapter 4

Epidemiology of Celiac Disease

Rahma Al Kindi, Asma Al Salmani, Rahma Al Hadhrami and Maryam Al Maashani

Abstract

Celiac disease (CD) is a chronic autoimmune disorder of the small bowel that is triggered by exposure to dietary gluten. In paediatric, CD commonly presents with intestinal manifestations, while in adults, many present with more subtle symptoms and extraintestinal manifestations, such as anaemia, fatigue, dermatitis, and headaches. The main scope of this chapter is to explore and present the prevalence of CD worldwide as well as trends in diagnosis over recent years. The prevalence of CD is approximately 0.5–1% in different regions of the world. However, exact prevalence rates may vary substantially in specific populations. Although CD was formerly believed to affect solely individuals of European ancestry, more recent studies indicate that the disease may have been either under-reported or undiagnosed in other populations. Moreover, it is possible that the increasing popularity of Western dietary practices may have an impact on the recent trend of increased rates of CD in non-Western populations. Certain population groups are also at high risk of developing CD, including first- or second-degree relatives of individuals with CD and those with diabetes or autoimmune disorders. Serological screening and HLA typing are therefore highly recommended for asymptomatic children in whom such risk factors are present.

Keywords: celiac disease, gluten, epidemiology, diagnosis, celiac disease trends

1. Introduction

Celiac disease (CD), also known as gluten-sensitive enteropathy, is a chronic autoimmune disorder characterised by mucosal inflammation of the small intestine, villous atrophy, and crypt hyperplasia. It is triggered by exposure to dietary gluten and related proteins in genetically susceptible individuals [1]. Gluten is the major protein found in cereals, including wheat, rye, and barley, and possibly oats [2]. Manifestations of CD are typically classified as either intestinal or extraintestinal. Common intestinal manifestations include diarrhoea or constipation, loss of appetite and weight, bloating, flatulence, abdominal pain, and nausea/vomiting [3]. However, many patients may present with extraintestinal manifestations, such as anaemia, fatigue, loss of bone density, dermatitis, ulcers, and headaches [3, 4].

Because CD can have such a heterogenous and vague clinical presentation, in which some manifestations may present at different ages or overlap with other, unrelated disorders, many individuals often go undiagnosed [4]. Human leukocyte antigen (HLA) tests are utilised as markers of CD, as approximately 98% of individuals with CD are either HLA-DQ2- or HLA-DQ8-positive [5]. For a definitive diagnosis, an upper oesophagogastroduodenoscopy with a small bowel biopsy should be performed for any patients with positive serology or for those with a high probability of having the disease (>5%), regardless of serology results [6]. The main intervention for CD is a lifelong commitment to a gluten-free diet.

2. Epidemiology

The prevalence of CD has been estimated to range from 0.5–1% in different parts of the world [7]. Mass screening for CD in four general European populations revealed a prevalence of 1% [8]. On the other hand, information regarding the prevalence of CD in the Middle East and among Arab populations is scarce and primarily based on small-scale studies [9]. Interestingly, research shows that there is an increased prevalence of CD among women compared to men, with a male-to-female ratio of 1:2.8, thereby indicating that women are diagnosed two to three times more frequently than men, [10–12] except in the young and elderly in which there is a more equal sex distribution [13]. However, in population-based screening studies, males and females appear more evenly affected, [14, 15] suggesting either gender-based differences in the severity of symptoms or in terms of access to health care. Indeed, a previous study has shown that men demonstrate greater evidence of severe illness at presentation compared to women [12].

Historically, CD was believed to be limited only to Europeans or people of European origin (i.e., North Americans and Caucasian Australians); however, advances in the availability of serological testing for CD—for instance, anti-gliadin antibody (AGA), anti-endomysial antibody (AEMA), and anti-transglutaminase antibody assays—have shown that CD is common not only in those of European ethnicity, but also those originating from developing countries in which the major dietary staple is wheat [16, 17]. Epidemiological research conducted in areas thought to be free of CD, including the Middle East, South Asia, Africa, and South America, has indicated that the disease was previously under-diagnosed in these regions [18].

The recent increase in the frequency of CD diagnoses in these areas can be also explained by growing uptake of Western breastfeeding and dietary practices (i.e., either short-lived or absence of breastfeeding and early weaning in infanthood combined with a greater amount of gluten intake thereafter). This suggests that many individuals may have a genetic predisposition to CD, but that clinical presentation only occurs when there is sufficient gluten present in the diet [13]. Because CD is the result of an interaction between both genetic (with regards to both HLA- and non-HLA-associated genes) and environmental factors (i.e., exposure to and levels of consumption of gluten-containing grains), it would be reasonable to evaluate the global distribution of these two components in order to identify specific areas and populations at risk for CD [19].

2.1 Europe

Several epidemiological studies performed in Italy have indicated that the prevalence of CD ranges from 0.2% to 0.74% [20–23]. However, studies from other European nations, including the United Kingdom, Sweden, Finland, and the

Netherlands have reported slightly higher prevalence rates, ranging from 1.0% to 2.0% [24–29].

2.2 North America

In the United States, the prevalence of adult CD is believed to be 0.95%, a rate similar to that reported in Europe, whereas the prevalence of paediatric CD has been calculated at 0.31%, with an overall prevalence ranging from 0.69% to 0.75% [14, 30, 31]. However, the prevalence of CD increases to 1.01% among non-Hispanic whites, with blacks and Hispanics in the United States showing considerably lower rates of CD at 0.3% and 0.2%, respectively [30, 32].

2.3 South America

The prevalence of CD in South America varies considerably between countries, despite their geographic proximity. In general, the prevalence of CD among Latin Americans is similar to that reported in Europeans. Overall, CD in Latin American populations is frequent and is primarily reported in populations and regions with Caucasian ancestry. Nevertheless, in certain countries with substantial Caucasian ancestry, such as Uruguay, the exact prevalence of CD remains unknown [33]. Studies conducted in Brazil have reported a prevalence of 1.5% in healthy blood donors [34, 35]. In an urban area of Argentina, the overall prevalence rate of CD among 2000 adults in the general population was 1:167, with the prevalence in women double that of men [36].

2.4 North Africa

In African populations, specifically in the Northern region of Africa, including Morocco, Algeria, Tunisia, Libya, and Egypt, the incidence of CD is very high and the disorder has been reported both in the general population and among at-risk groups [37–39]. Serological screening of 2500 Tunisian healthy blood donors showed that the prevalence of AEMAs in the general population was 1:355, which is close to that of Europeans. These high frequencies are not surprising given that wheat and barley are major staple foods in these countries and because there is high frequency of the HLA-DR3/DQ2 CD-predisposing haplotypes in these populations [38].

Another population in North Africa with an elevated prevalence of CD is the Saharawi people native to the western part of the Sahara desert; these individuals, many of whom live as refugees in Algeria, are of Arab and Berber origin and traditionally show a high degree of consanguinity. The elevated prevalence of CD in this population may be explained both by genetic factors, as the Saharawi population has a very high frequency of the HLA-DR3/DQ2 haplotype, and by environmental factors, because of changes in their dietary habits over the last few decades. For example, rates and duration of breastfeeding have been reduced and large amounts of gluten are now being consumed by infants and children in early life as part of their staple diet, due to food aid being supplied by Western countries as part of ongoing humanitarian programmes [40].

2.5 Asia

In the Asian Pacific islands (i.e., Indonesia, South Korea, and the Philippines), CD is likely to be rare because of the low wheat consumption in these populations and the low frequency of the HLA-DQB1*02 haplotype. In turn, in Southeast Asia, the HLA-DQB1*02 haplotype is often present in more than 5% of the population, but CD is nevertheless still predicted to be rare, as staple diets are traditionally based on rice [41]. In China, CD was previously thought to be uncommon; however, recent serological testing of adolescents and young adults in areas in which wheat is a dietary staple has indicated that the prevalence of the disorder may be as high as 0.76% [42].

2.6 The Middle East

Until the 1990s, CD was considered to be very rare in the Middle East. However, with the introduction of AEA and AGA testing, CD has been more readily reported from developing Middle Eastern countries at a rate similar to that of Western countries [43–46]. However, this prevalence varies from 0.6% to 1.17% in low-risk populations, and from 2.4–19% in high-risk populations [47]. The prevalence of CD in Middle Eastern countries among low-risk populations is similar to that reported in Western countries, but is higher in high-risk populations, such as those with type 1 diabetes mellitus (T1DM). The frequency of the disorder is likely underestimated because of the lack of clinical suspicion and low patient awareness of the disease and its symptoms in this region of the world [47].

3. Trends over recent years

Over the last 50 years, the incidence of CD has steadily risen, and this may be only in part attributed to heightened clinician awareness and the advent of serological studies that can detect cases of what used to be subclinical disease. Environmental factors, such as gluten intake in infanthood, infections, and socioeconomic status may also play a role [48]. Serological screening studies have shown a dramatic increase in CD serology positivity over time [49–52]. In a study by Rubio-Tapia *et al.*, the researchers reported a four- to five-fold increase in CD over 50 years; [28] in addition, the prevalence of the disease appears to increase with age from 1% in children to 2.45% among an elderly cohort in Finland [28, 52].

Nonetheless, it remains true that the bulk of those with CD continue to go undiagnosed [24, 53]. Moreover, the rate of diagnosis varies in different countries, with a high in Finland in which about 70% of those with CD are diagnosed, [54] compared to the United States in which only 5% are diagnosed [53]. However, even within the United States, the rate of diagnosis has begun increasing in both adults and children [55, 56].

4. Risk groups

The prevalence of CD, as detected by screening programmes using specific antibodies, is substantially increased in several risk groups as compared with the general population. High-risk groups for CD include: first-degree relatives of individuals with CD (range: 5% to 7.5%), second-degree relatives of individuals with CD (range: 2–3%), and individuals with T1DM (range: 5–10%), Down syndrome (range: 5–12%), or autoimmune thyroid disease (range: 2–7%); in addition, CD is also associated with Turner syndrome (range: 4–8%), Williams syndrome, and selective immunoglobulin

A deficiency (each with 8% risk) [14, 57–63]. Thus, because of their increased risk, routine screening for CD is recommended in asymptomatic children with these conditions.

The overall prevalence of CD is highly dependent on HLA-DQ2/DQ8 typing and gluten consumption. Individuals with positive HLA typing for CD have a high chance of developing symptoms when consuming high amounts of gluten. Moreover, those with diabetes, autoimmune disorders, or who are relatives of individuals with CD have an even higher risk of developing CD, since they also share the same HLA typing [7].

5. Conclusions

Globally, the prevalence of CD ranges from approximately 0.5–1% in different regions of the world. However, exact prevalence rates may vary substantially in specific populations. Although CD was formerly believed to affect solely individuals of European ancestry, more recent studies indicate that the disease may have been either under-reported or undiagnosed in other populations. Moreover, it is possible that the increasing popularity of Western breastfeeding and dietary practices may have an impact on the recent trend of increased rates of CD in non-Western populations. Certain population groups are also at high risk of developing CD, including first- or second-degree relatives of individuals with CD and those with diabetes or autoimmune disorders. Serological screening and HLA typing are therefore highly recommended for asymptomatic children in whom such risk factors are present.

Conflict of interest

The authors declare no conflicts of interest.

Abbreviations

AEMA	anti-endomysial antibody
AGA	anti-gliadin antibody
CD	celiac disease
HLA	human leukocyte antigen
T1DM	Type 1 diabetes mellitus

Author details

Rahma Al Kindi[1*], Asma Al Salmani[1], Rahma Al Hadhrami[1]
and Maryam Al Maashani[2]

1 Department of Family Medicine and Public Health, Sultan Qaboos University Hospital, Muscat, Oman

2 Directorate General of Health Services, Taqah Hospital, Dhofar, Oman

*Address all correspondence to: alrahma23@gmail.com

References

[1] Rostom A, Dubé C, Cranney A, Saloojee N, Sy R, Garritty C, et al. Celiac disease: Summary. In: AHRQ Evidence Report Summaries. Rockville: Agency for Healthcare Research and Quality; 2004. p. 04-E029-1

[2] Malalgoda M, Simsek S. Celiac disease and cereal proteins. Food Hydrocolloids. 2017;**68**:108-113. DOI: 10.1016/j.foodhyd.2016.09.024

[3] Caio G, Volta U, Sapone A, Leffler DA, De Giorgio R, Catassi C, et al. Celiac disease: A comprehensive current review. BMC Medicine. 2019;**17**:142. DOI: 10.1186/s12916-019-1380-z

[4] Laurikka P, Nurminen S, Kivelä L, Kurppa K. Extraintestinal manifestations of celiac disease: Early detection for better long-term outcomes. Nutrients. 2018;**10**:1015. DOI: 10.3390/nu10081015

[5] Case S, Adams PC. Celiac disease – Hidden and dangerous. Canadian Journal of Gastroenterology. 2006;**20**:571-573. DOI: 10.1155/2006/748649

[6] Casella S, Zanini B, Lanzarotto F, Villanacci V, Ricci C, Lanzini A. Celiac disease in elderly adults: Clinical, serological, and histological characteristics and the effect of a gluten-free diet. Journal of the American Geriatrics Society. 2012;**60**:1064-1069. DOI: 10.1111/j.1532-5415.2012.03997.x

[7] Gujral N, Freeman HJ, Thomson ABR. Celiac disease: Prevalence, diagnosis, pathogenesis and treatment. World Journal of Gastroenterology. 2012;**18**:6036-6059. DOI: 10.3748/wjg.v18.i42.6036

[8] Mustalahti K, Catassi C, Reunanen A, Fabiani E, Heier M, McMillan S, et al. The prevalence of celiac disease in Europe: Results of a centralized, international mass screening project. Annals of Medicine. 2010;**42**:587-595. DOI: 10.3109/07853890.2010.505931

[9] Saadah OI. Celiac disease in children and adolescents at a single center in Saudi Arabia. Annals of Saudi Medicine. 2011;**31**:51-57. DOI: 10.4103/0256-4947.75779

[10] Thomas HJ, Ahmad T, Rajaguru C, Barnardo M, Warren BF, Jewell DP. Contribution of histological, serological, and genetic factors to the clinical heterogeneity of adult-onset coeliac disease. Scandinavian Journal of Gastroenterology. 2009;**44**:1076-1083. DOI: 10.1080/00365520903100473

[11] Hin H, Bird G, Fisher P, Mahy N, Jewell D. Coeliac disease in primary care: Case finding study. BMJ. 1999;**318**:164-167. DOI: 10.1136/bmj.318.7177.164

[12] Bai D, Brar P, Holleran S, Ramakrishnan R, Green PHR. Effect of gender on the manifestations of celiac disease: Evidence for greater malabsorption in men. Scandinavian Journal of Gastroenterology. 2005;**40**:183-187. DOI: 10.1080/00365520510011498

[13] Green PHR, Stavropoulos SN, Panagi SG, Goldstein SL, McMahon DJ, Absan H, et al. Characteristics of adult celiac disease in the USA: Results of a national survey. The American Journal of Gastroenterology. 2001;**96**:126-131. DOI: 10.1111/j.1572-0241.2001.03462.x

[14] Fasano A, Berti I, Gerarduzzi T, Not T, Colletti RB, Drago S, et al. Prevalence of celiac disease in at-risk and not-at-risk groups in the United States:

A large multicenter study. Archives of Internal Medicine. 2003;**163**:286-292. DOI: 10.1001/archinte.163.3.286

[15] Katz KD, Rashtak S, Lahr BD, Melton LJ 3rd, Krause PK, Maggi K, et al. Screening for celiac disease in a North American population: Sequential serology and gastrointestinal symptoms. The American Journal of Gastroenterology. 2011;**106**:1333-1339. DOI: 10.1038/ajg.2011.21

[16] Sher KS, Fraser RC, Wicks AC, Mayberry JF. High risk of coeliac disease in Punjabis. Epidemiological study in the south Asian and European populations of Leicestershire. Digestion. 1993;**54**:178-182. DOI: 10.1159/000201035

[17] Cataldo F, Montalto G. Celiac disease in the developing countries: A new and challenging public health problem. World Journal of Gastroenterology. 2007;**13**:2153-2159. DOI: 10.3748/wjg.v13.i15.2153

[18] Catassi C, Yachha SK. The global village of celiac disease. In: Fasano A, Troncone R, Branski D, editors. Frontiers in Celiac Disease. Vol. 12. Basel: Karger; 2008. pp. 23-31. DOI: 10.1159/000128610

[19] Fasano A, Catassi C. Current approaches to diagnosis and treatment of celiac disease: An evolving spectrum. Gastroenterology. 2001;**120**:636-651. DOI: 10.1053/gast.2001.22123

[20] Tommasini A, Not T, Kiren V, Baldas V, Santon D, Trevisiol C, et al. Mass screening for coeliac disease using antihuman transglutaminase antibody assay. Archives of Disease in Childhood. 2004;**89**:512-515. DOI: 10.1136/adc.2003.029603

[21] Catassi C, Fanciulli G, D'Appello AR, El Asmar R, Rondina C, Fabiani E, et al. Antiendomysium versus antigliadin antibodies in screening the general population for coeliac disease. Scandinavian Journal of Gastroenterology. 2000;**35**:732-736. DOI: 10.1080/003655200750023408

[22] Trevisiol C, Not T, Berti I, Buratti E, Città A, Neri E, et al. Screening for coeliac disease in healthy blood donors at two immuno-transfusion centres in north-East Italy. Italian Journal of Gastroenterology and Hepatology. 1999;**31**:584-586

[23] Volta U, Bellentani S, Bianchi FB, Brandi G, De Franceschi L, Miglioli L, et al. High prevalence of celiac disease in Italian general population. Digestive Diseases and Sciences. 2001;**46**:1500-1505. DOI: 10.1023/a:1010648122797

[24] West J, Logan RFA, Hill PG, Lloyd A, Lewis S, Hubbard R, et al. Seroprevalence, correlates, and characteristics of undetected coeliac disease in England. Gut. 2003;**52**:960-965. DOI: 10.1136/gut.52.7.960

[25] Carlsson AK, Axelsson IE, Borulf SK, Bredberg AC, Ivarsson SA. Serological screening for celiac disease in healthy 2.5-year-old children in Sweden. Pediatrics. 2001;**107**:42-45. DOI: 10.1542/peds.107.1.42

[26] Walker MM, Murray JA, Ronkainen J, Aro P, Storskrubb T, D'Amato M, et al. Detectionofceliacdiseaseandlymphocytic enteropathy by parallel serology and histopathology in a population-based study. Gastroenterology. 2010;**139**:112-119. DOI: 10.1053/j.gastro.2010.04.007

[27] Kolho KL, Färkkilä MA, Savilahti E. Undiagnosed coeliac disease is common in Finnish adults. Scandinavian Journal of Gastroenterology. 1998;**33**:1280-1283. DOI: 10.1080/00365529850172368

[28] Mäki M, Mustalahti K, Kokkonen J, Kulmala P, Haapalahti M, Karttunen T,

et al. Prevalence of celiac disease among children in Finland. The New England Journal of Medicine. 2003;**348**:2517-2524. DOI: 10.1056/NEJMoa021687

[29] Csizmadia CG, Mearin ML, von Blomberg BM, Brand R, Verloove-Vanhorick SP. An iceberg of childhood coeliac disease in the Netherlands. Lancet. 1999;**353**:813-814. DOI: 10.1016/S0140-6736(99)00243-3

[30] Rubio-Tapia A, Ludvigsson JF, Brantner TL, Murray JA, Everhart JE. The prevalence of celiac disease in the United States. The American Journal of Gastroenterology. 2012;**107**:1538-1544. DOI: 10.1038/ajg.2012.219

[31] Kim HS, Patel KG, Orosz E, Kothari N, Demyen MF, Pyrsopoulos N, et al. Time trends in the prevalence of celiac disease and gluten-free diet in the US population: Results from the National Health and Nutrition Examination Surveys 2009-2014. JAMA Internal Medicine. 2016;**176**:1716-1717. DOI: 10.1001/jamainternmed.2016.5254

[32] Choung RS, Ditah IC, Nadeau AM, Rubio-Tapia A, Marietta EV, Brantner TL, et al. Trends and racial/ ethnic disparities in gluten-sensitive problems in the United States: Findings from the National Health and Nutrition Examination Surveys from 1988 to 2012. The American Journal of Gastroenterology. 2015;**110**:455-461. DOI: 10.1038/ajg.2015.8

[33] Parra-Medina R, Molano-Gonzalez N, Rojas-Villarraga A, Agmon-Levin N, Arango MT, Shoenfeld Y, et al. Prevalence of celiac disease in Latin America: A systematic review and meta-regression. PLoS One. 2015;**10**:e0124040. DOI: 10.1371/journal.pone.0124040

[34] Gandolfi L, Pratesi R, Cordoba JC, Tauil PL, Gasparin M, Catassi C. Prevalence of celiac disease among blood donors in Brazil. The American Journal of Gastroenterology. 2000;**95**:689-692. DOI: 10.1111/j.1572-0241.2000.01847.x

[35] Oliveira RP, Sdepanian VL, Barreto JA, Cortez AJP, Carvalho FO, Bordin JO, et al. High prevalence of celiac disease in Brazilian blood donor volunteers based on screening by IgA antitissue transglutaminase antibody. European Journal of Gastroenterology & Hepatology. 2007;**19**:43-49. DOI: 10.1097/01.meg.0000250586.61232.a3

[36] Gomez JC, Selvaggio GS, Viola M, Pizarro B, la Motta G, de Barrio S, et al. Prevalence of celiac disease in Argentina: Screening of an adult population in the La Plata area. The American Journal of Gastroenterology. 2001;**96**:2700-2704. DOI: 10.1111/j.1572-0241.2001.04124.x

[37] Ashabani A, Errabtea H, Shapan A, Tuckova L, Tlaskalova-Hogenova H. Serologic markers of untreated celiac disease in Libyan children: Antigliadin, antitransglutaminase, antiendomysial, and anticalreticulin antibodies. Journal of Pediatric Gastroenterology and Nutrition. 2001;**33**:276-282. DOI: 10.1097/00005176-200109000-00009

[38] Mankaï A, Landolsi H, Chahed A, Gueddah L, Limem M, Ben Abdessalem M, et al. Celiac disease in Tunisia: Serological screening in healthy blood donors. Pathological Biology (Paris). 2006;**54**:10-13. DOI: 10.1016/j.patbio.2005.02.005

[39] Catassi C, Abu-Zakry M, Kryszak D, Fasano A. Abstract: Celiac disease among schoolchildren in Egypt: Results of a pilot study. In: Proceedings of the 2004 11th International Symposium on Coeliac Disease. Belfast: University of Maryland Baltimore; 2004, 2004

[40] Lionetti P, Favilli T, Chiaravalloti G, Ughi C, Maggiore G. Coeliac disease in

Saharawi children in Algerian refugee camps. Lancet. 1999;**353**:1189-1190. DOI: 10.1016/S0140-6736(05)74414-7

[41] Cummins AG, Roberts-Thomson IC. Prevalence of celiac disease in the Asia-Pacific region. Journal of Gastroenterology and Hepatology. 2009;**24**:1347-1351. DOI: 10.1111/j. 1440-1746.2009.05932.x

[42] Yuan J, Zhou C, Gao J, Li J, Yu F, Lu J, et al. Prevalence of celiac disease autoimmunity among adolescents and young adults in China. Clinical Gastroenterology and Hepatology. 2017;**15**:1572-1579.e1. DOI: 10.1016/j. cgh.2017.04.025

[43] Rostami K, Malekzadeh R, Shahbazkhani B, Akbari MR, Catassi C. CoeliacdiseaseinMiddleEasterncountries: A challenge for the evolutionary history of this complex disorder? Digestive and Liver Disease. 2004;**36**:694-697. DOI: 10.1016/j.dld.2004.05.010

[44] Gursoy S, Guven K, Simsek T, Yurci A, Torun E, Koc N, et al. The prevalence of unrecognized adult celiac disease in Central Anatolia. Journal of Clinical Gastroenterology. 2005;**39**:508-511. DOI: 10.1097/01. mcg.0000165664.87153.e1

[45] Tatar G, Elsurer R, Simsek H, Balaban YH, Hascelik G, Ozcebe OI, et al. Screening of tissue transglutaminase antibody in healthy blood donors for celiac disease screening in the Turkish population. Digestive Diseases and Sciences. 2004;**49**:1479-1484. DOI: 10.1023/b:ddas.0000042250.59327.91

[46] Akbari MR, Mohammadkhani A, Fakheri H, Zahedi MJ, Shahbazkhani B, Nouraie M, et al. Screening of the adult population in Iran for coeliac disease: Comparison of the tissue-transglutaminase antibody and anti-endomysial antibody tests. European Journal of Gastroenterology & Hepatology. 2006;**18**:1181-1186. DOI: 10.1097/01.meg.0000224477. 51428.32

[47] Barada K, Bitar A, Mokadem MAR, Hashash JG, Green P. Celiac disease in Middle Eastern and North African countries: A new burden? World Journal of Gastroenterology. 2010;**16**:1449-1457. DOI: 10.3748/wjg.v16.i12.1449

[48] Tack GJ, Verbeek WHM, Schreurs MWJ, Mulder CJJ. The spectrum of celiac disease: Epidemiology, clinical aspects and treatment. Nature Reviews. Gastroenterology & Hepatology. 2010;7:204-213. DOI: 10.1038/ nrgastro.2010.23

[49] Lohi S, Mustalahti K, Kaukinen K, Laurila K, Collin P, Rissanen H, et al. Increasing prevalence of coeliac disease over time. Alimentary Pharmacology & Therapeutics. 2007;**26**:1217-1225. DOI: 10.1111/j.1365-2036.2007.03502.x

[50] Vilppula A, Kaukinen K, Luostarinen L, Krekelä I, Patrikainen H, Valve R, et al. Increasing prevalence and high incidence of celiac disease in elderly people: A population-based study. BMC Gastroenterology. 2009;**9**:49. DOI: 10.1186/1471-230X-9-49

[51] Vilppula A, Collin P, Mäki M, Valve R, Luostarinen M, Krekelä I, et al. Undetected coeliac disease in the elderly: A biopsy-proven population-based study. Digestive and Liver Disease. 2008;**40**:809-813. DOI: 10.1016/j. dld.2008.03.013

[52] Rubio-Tapia A, Kyle RA, Kaplan EL, Johnson DR, Page W, Erdtmann F, et al. Increased prevalence and mortality in undiagnosed celiac disease. Gastroenterology. 2009;**137**:88-93. DOI: 10.1053/j.gastro.2009.03.059

[53] Murray JA, Van Dyke C, Plevak MF, Dierkhising RA, Zinsmeister AR, Melton LJ 3rd. Trends in the identification and clinical features of celiac disease in a North American community, 1950-2001. Clinical Gastroenterology and Hepatology. 2003;**1**:19-27. DOI: 10.1053/jcgh.2003.50004

[54] Collin P, Huhtala H, Virta L, Kekkonen L, Reunala T. Diagnosis of celiac disease in clinical practice: Physician's alertness to the condition essential. Journal of Clinical Gastroenterology. 2007;**41**:152-156. DOI: 10.1097/01.mcg.0000212618.12455.a8

[55] Green PHR, Neugut AI, Naiyer AJ, Edwards ZC, Gabinelle S, Chinburapa V. Economic benefits of increased diagnosis of celiac disease in a national managed care population in the United States. Journal of Insurance Medicine. 2008;**40**:218-228

[56] Telega G, Bennet TR, Werlin S. Emerging new clinical patterns in the presentation of celiac disease. Archives of Pediatrics & Adolescent Medicine. 2008;**162**:164-168. DOI: 10.1001/archpediatrics.2007.38

[57] Hill ID, Dirks MH, Liptak GS, Colletti RB, Fasano A, Guandalini S, et al. Guideline for the diagnosis and treatment of celiac disease in children: Recommendations of the north American Society for Pediatric Gastroenterology, Hepatology and nutrition. Journal of Pediatric Gastroenterology and Nutrition. 2005;**40**:1-19. DOI: 10.1097/00005176-200501000-00001

[58] Hoffenberg EJ, Bao F, Eisenbarth GS, Uhlhorn C, Haas JE, Sokol RJ, et al. Transglutaminase antibodies in children with a genetic risk for celiac disease. The Journal of Pediatrics. 2000;**137**:356-360. DOI: 10.1067/mpd.2000.107582

[59] Hummel M, Bonifacio E, Stern M, Dittler J, Schimmel A, Ziegler AG. Development of celiac disease-associated antibodies in offspring of parents with type I diabetes. Diabetologia. 2000;**43**:1005-1011. DOI: 10.1007/s001250051483

[60] Crone J, Rami B, Huber WD, Granditsch G, Schober E. Prevalence of celiac disease and follow-up of EMA in children and adolescents with type 1 diabetes mellitus. Journal of Pediatric Gastroenterology and Nutrition. 2003;**37**:67-71. DOI: 10.1097/00005176-200307000-00011

[61] Bonamico M, Pasquino AM, Mariani P, Danesi HM, Culasso F, Mazzanti L, et al. Prevalence and clinical picture of celiac disease in turner syndrome. The Journal of Clinical Endocrinology and Metabolism. 2002;**87**:5495-5498. DOI: 10.1210/jc.2002-020855

[62] Giannotti A, Tiberio G, Castro M, Virgilii F, Colistro F, Ferretti F, et al. Coeliac disease in Williams syndrome. Journal of Medical Genetics. 2001;**38**:767-768. DOI: 10.1136/jmg.38.11.767

[63] Størdal K, Bakken IJ, Surén P, Stene LC. Epidemiology of coeliac disease and comorbidity in Norwegian children. Journal of Pediatric Gastroenterology and Nutrition. 2013;**57**:467-471. DOI: 10.1097/MPG.0b013e3182a455dd

Chapter 5

The Role of the Gluten-Free Diet in the Development of Malignancies in Celiac Disease

Maiara Botosso, Renatta Damasceno and Priscila Farage

Abstract

Celiac disease (CD) is an autoimmune disorder that can lead to serious health consequences, including cancer. The gluten-free diet (GFD) is the primary treatment for CD and has been shown to lead to clinical remission of the disease. However, the effect of the GFD on cancer development in CD patients is not well understood. This narrative review analyzed observational studies investigating the association between cancer development and adherence to the GFD in CD patients. The most common cancer identified was non-Hodgkin's lymphoma, followed by others such as colon carcinoma and thyroid cancer. Late diagnosis, type of cancer, and type of CD were factors relevant to the protective role of the GFD. However, there is still no consensus in the scientific literature regarding the GFD's role in cancer development in CD. While some studies suggest a protective role, others have not identified an association between the GFD and cancer. More research is needed to understand the relationship between the GFD and cancer development in CD patients. Nonetheless, the GFD is essential for the clinical, serological, and histological remission of CD and improved quality of life.

Keywords: celiac disease, malignancy, cancer, gluten-free diet, gluten

1. Introduction

Celiac disease (CD) is an autoimmune systemic disorder with multiple clinical manifestations triggered by the ingestion of gluten in genetically predisposed individuals [1]. The only available effective treatment so far consists of excluding gluten-protein fractions found in wheat, rye, barley, and hybrids like kamut and triticale—from the diet [2]. CD may occur at all ages and present a variety of signs and symptoms such as stunted growth/short stature, weight loss, abdominal pain, diarrhea/constipation, irritability, osteoporosis, iron-deficiency anemia, among others [3]. Moreover, CD has been associated with increased mortality due to long-term complications such as lymphoproliferative malignancy [4].

Cancer is defined as a chronic multifactorial disease characterized by the uncontrolled growth of cells, and it represents the second leading cause of death worldwide, with the expectation that the number of cases will increase significantly in the coming decades [5, 6]. One of the most serious possible complications of CD is the development of malignancies. In a retrospective population-based cohort in Sweden, Lebwohl et al. [4]

evaluated the association between CD and mortality risk in 49.829 patients compared to control participants in the general population matched by age, sex, county and calendar period (n = 246.426). The authors found that CD patients displayed increased risk of death from cancer (2.7 vs. 2.2 per 1000 person-years; HR, 1.29 [95% CI, 1.22–1.36]).

The precise risk of malignancy in adult celiac patients is difficult to assess. However, studies indicate that untreated patients with severe histological intestinal damage are more susceptible to developing cancer [2]. In the retrospective cohort study by Ludvigsson et al. [7], the mortality in CD was examined according to small-intestinal histopathology. The authors identified the highest hazard ratio (HR) in the first year after biopsy with an HR of 3.78 for death due to malignancy (95% CI, 3.14–4.55). After 5 years of follow-up, death from malignancy was only moderately increased (HR, 1.17; 95% CI, 1.03–1.33), which might be explained by the longer duration of treatment at this point, as mucosal inflammation may persist up to a year after implementation of the gluten-free diet (GFD).

The benefits of the GFD on the health and clinical manifestations of CD patients are well established in the literature. A large proportion of these individuals respond completely to the GFD and have a normal life expectancy. However, variables such as late diagnosis, advanced age and low adherence to the GFD represent risk factors for the development of disease complications [8]. Although it may seem simple to remove gluten from the diet, CD treatment may be compromised due to lack of widespread availability of gluten-free products, their high cost, the risk of cross-contamination, the social burden caused by the restrictive nature of the diet, among other factors. Together, these variables may lead to low adherence to the GFD [9].

In a recent study, Marafini, Monteleone and Stolfi [10] suggested that since non-adherence or non-responsiveness to the GFD may lead to chronic inflammation of the small intestine, it is tempting to speculate that a gluten-containing diet in celiac patients could promote the activation of immune/inflammatory signals and ultimately favor the onset or progression of lymphomas and intestinal carcinomas.

Although CD is a common condition with potentially serious health consequences, including cancer, very few studies specifically address the GFD as a possible protective factor in the development of malignancies in celiac individuals. Therefore, this narrative review discusses the role of the GFD in the onset of malignancies in CD, prevalence and characteristics of the main types of cancer found in these patients and the importance of the diet to the treatment and prevention of complications.

2. Methods

The literature search was carried out in 2022 and updated in 2023 for articles that analyzed the role of the GFD in the development of malignancies in patients with CD. No time restrictions were applied for publication date. The following electronic databases were used: Scielo (Scientific Electronic Library Online), Lilacs (Latin American and Caribbean Centre on Health Sciences Information), Pubmed (US National Library of Medicine—National Institutes of Health), Google Scholar and the Brazilian Digital Library of Theses and Dissertations. The search was conducted by two researchers independently and without conflicts of interest.

The keywords used were "coeliac/celiac disease", "cancer", "malignancy", "neoplasm", "lymphoma", "gluten-free diet", "dietary adherence", and corresponding terms in Portuguese and Spanish. The Boolean operators AND and OR were used to combine the descriptors.

Original articles (observational studies: cross-sectional, case control and cohort) that investigated a possible association between the occurrence of malignancies and adherence or not to a GFD in patients with CD were included in this review. The following exclusion criteria were applied: (i) reviews, letters, conference summaries, case reports and books; (ii) studies that did not evaluate the GFD in the context of cancer development and (iii) studies that did not follow the criteria recommended by the European Society for Paediatric Gastroenterology Hepatology and Nutrition for the diagnosis of CD (characteristic mucosal changes observed by intestinal biopsy and serological testing).

For the selection of articles, all the abstracts were read and the ones that met the inclusion criteria were chosen. Studies were analyzed according to the year of publication, origin country, aim, study design, sample characterization, main results and conclusions regarding the role of the GFD in the onset of cancer in patients with CD.

3. Results and discussion

After reading, analyzing and excluding studies that did not meet the established criteria, eight articles were selected to compose this review (**Figure 1**).

The general characteristics and main data of the studies are described in **Table 1**.

The articles included in this review were published between 2003 and 2014. One study was conducted in Argentina, one is from the United States, one from Sweden, and five are from Italy. Regarding the design of the studies, four were prospective cohorts, two retrospective cohorts, one case control and one retrospective case control. All screened articles were extracted from the PubMed database and written in English.

The American study by Green et al. [11] aimed to estimate the risk of malignancy in a cohort of patients with CD compared to the general population of the United States and to determine whether a GFD would be protective in this regard.

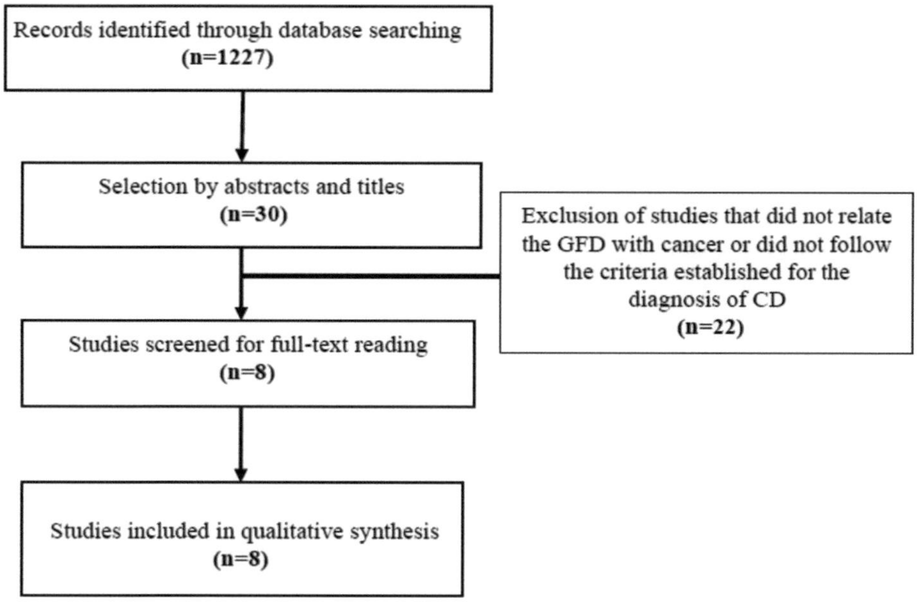

Figure 1.
Flow diagram of literature search and selection criteria.

Author/ year	Study design	Country	Aim	Sample (n)	Main results	Conclusion
[11]	Prospective cohort	United States of America	To estimate the risk of malignancy in a cohort of patients with celiac disease compared to the general US population and to determine whether a gluten-free diet is protective.	381 patients from the New York Presbyterian Hospital (245 women and 136 men).	In CD patients, an increased risk of small bowel adenocarcinoma, esophageal cancer, melanoma and non-Hodgkin's lymphoma was observed compared to the general population.	Despite the increased risk of cancer in celiac patients, this is observed before the diagnosis of CD and may be reduced with strict adherence to a GFD. The risk for non-Hodgkin's lymphoma, however, appears to persist despite treatment with a GDF.
[12]	Prospective cohort	Italy	To estimate the risk of developing cancer in undiagnosed celiac patients and assess whether this risk correlates with the age of patients at the time of CD diagnosis.	1968 patients (1485 women and 483 men/ mean age = 36.2 years) diagnosed with CD at collaborating centers of the Italian Registry of Celiac Disease Complications.	This study suggests that the GFD probably protects against the development of malignancies in CD patients, since the older the age at CD diagnosis, the greater the risk of cancer.	The GFD is probably protective against the development of malignancies in CD patients.
[13]	Prospective cohort	Italy	To assess whether strict adherence to a GFD reduces the risk of developing enteropathy-associated T-cell lymphoma.	1757 patients (443 men and 1314 women/ mean age = 38.6 years) diagnosed with CD at collaborating centers of the Italian Registry of Celiac Disease Complications.	The risk of developing intestinal lymphoma in celiac patients who maintain gluten in the diet was significantly higher compared to the risk in patients who followed the diet properly.	These results show that a GFD is protective against the development of CD-associated T-cell lymphoma.
[14]	Retrospective cohort	Italy	To evaluate the incidence of malignant and non-malignant complications in a cohort of patients with CD on a GFD, and to assess whether the onset of complications is related to non-adherence to the diet.	549 patients (no further sample details).	A total of 3.3% of patients developed complications on a GFD (n = 18), with 7 of them being malignant and 11 non-malignant. Complications appear to be independent of optimal adherence to the GFD and seem to affect patients diagnosed with classic CD more than patients with subclinical CD.	In this study, no association was identified between adherence to a GFD and the onset of malignancies.

Author/ year	Study design	Country	Aim	Sample (n)	Main results	Conclusion
[15]	Case control	Sweden	To investigate the importance of CD features and adherence to a GFD for lymphoma risk.	59 lymphoma patients and 137 matched controls (n = 196) from a population cohort of 11,650 inpatients with CD. Out of the 196 participants, 81 were men and 115, women.	Low dietary adherence was not significantly associated with overall lymphoma risk (odds ratio 1.83, 95% confidence interval 0.78–4.31) or with lymphoma subtypes. There was, however, an indication of increased risk of B-cell lymphoma (odds ratio 4.74, confidence interval 0.89–25.3) or extra-intestinal lymphoma (odds ratio 3.00, confidence interval 0.73–12.3) in poor adherence to the diet.	Adherence to the GFD did not significantly alter lymphoma risk, but a moderate effect cannot be ruled out.
[16]	Prospective cohort	Italy	To carry out a prospective analysis of the risk of celiac patients developing thyroid carcinoma.	1757 patients (443 men and 1314 women/mean age = 38.6 years).	The number of dietary transgressions per month (frequency of consumption of gluten-containing foods) did not correlate with the development of thyroid carcinoma.	Strict adherence to a GFD does not seem to protect against the development of this malignancy.
[17]	Retrospective case control	Argentina	To determine the risk of colorectal neoplasia among patients with CD.	354 patients (118 cases and 236 controls). Patients with CD were considered cases and those without CD were considered controls. For each case, two controls were randomly selected and matched for age, gender, indication for colonoscopy and family history of first- and second-degree colorectal cancer.	The study did not indicate a greater risk of colorectal neoplasia in patients with CD, since the risk of polyps, adenomas and advanced neoplastic lesions was similar in both groups. In individuals with CD, poor adherence to the GFD was independently associated with the presence of adenomas (odds ratio 6.78, confidence interval 1.39–33.20 $p = 0.01$).	Low adherence to a GFD increases the risk of developing adenomas.

Author/ year	Study design	Country	Aim	Sample (n)	Main results	Conclusion
[18]	Retrospective cohort	Italy	To describe the risk of colon cancer in a group of celiac patients.	1757 patients (443 men and 1314 women).	During the study period, six patients developed colon carcinoma. The standardized incidence rate resulted in 0.29 (95% CI = 0.07–0.45). When the risk was stratified by gluten intake, the incidence rate dropped to 0.07 (95% CI = 0.009–0.27) for patients with strict adherence to the GFD.	The low risk of developing cancer in CD patients decreases during the first year after diagnosis and is even lower for celiac patients following a strict GFD.

Table 1.
Studies on the role of a gluten-free diet in the development of malignancies in celiac disease patients.

Participants were treated between July 1981 and January 2000 at the New York Presbyterian Hospital, which has a reference center for CD. Adherence to the GFD was questioned at the initial contact and at subsequent visits by an investigator, with no further details on the content of the questions. The frequency of conscious/voluntary gluten ingestion in the previous month was evaluated.

Among a total of 381 patients, 64% were women (n = 245). During the study period, 3.4% of participants died (n = 13), eight of them due to cancer. A total of 11.3% (n = 43) were diagnosed with malignancy: nine after CD diagnosis, seven within a month of diagnosis and 27 before diagnosis. The most common neoplasm identified was non-Hodgkin's lymphoma (NHL) (n = 9), followed by breast cancer (n = 5), melanoma (n = 5), small intestine (n = 3), colon (n = 3), esophagus (n = 3), lung (n = 3), chronic lymphocytic leukemia (n = 2), ovarian (n = 2) and cervical cancer (n = 2). The study results revealed an increased risk of malignancy in patients with CD compared to the general population of the United States. This finding is consistent with European studies that reported higher rates of cancer of the small intestine, esophagus and lymphoma among individuals with celiac disease [19].

It is important to emphasize that most of these cancer cases occurred before the diagnosis of CD, and a late diagnosis means longer exposure of the patient to dietary gluten. However, an increased risk of NHL was identified among participants despite their strict adherence to a GFD for about 5 years. Thus, the authors suggest that the increased risk for cancer in general occurs before the diagnosis of CD and that it may be reduced with compliance to the GFD. The risk of non-Hodgkin's lymphoma, however, appears to persist despite adequate dietary treatment [11].

In 2007, Silano and colleagues published a study which may be compared to the work by Green et al. [11]. The objective was to evaluate whether the late diagnosis of CD and the consequent prolonged dietary exposure to gluten would increase the risk of developing neoplasia. The study population consisted of patients diagnosed with CD at the Italian Gastroenterology Centers between January 1982 and March 2005. A total of 1968 individuals were included, of whom 1485 were women (75.4%), with a mean age at CD diagnosis of 36.2 ± 13.8 years [12].

Among 1968 patients, 55 were diagnosed with cancer (2.09%) either before or simultaneously with the diagnosis of CD, compared to 42.1 expected cases, with a standardized morbidity ratio (SMR) of 1.3 (95% CI = 1.0–1.7). The most frequent malignant neoplasm was gastrointestinal non-Hodgkin lymphoma (n = 20), followed by colon carcinoma (n = 7), adenocarcinoma of the small intestine (n = 5), Hodgkin lymphoma (n = 4) and stomach and breast carcinomas (n = 3). Other tumor locations included liver, lung, ovary, thyroid cancer and myeloma (two cases each) and acute leukemia, melanoma and uterus (one case each). No patient developed two or more cancers [12].

The mean age at CD diagnosis for patients who developed cancer was 47.6 ± 10.2 years, which was significantly higher than the age at CD diagnosis for patients who did not develop malignancies (28.6 ± 18.2 years). Therefore, this study suggests that the GFD is a likely protector against the development of malignancies in CD patients, as the older the age at CD diagnosis, the longer the exposure time to gluten and the higher the risk of cancer [12].

Enteropathy-associated T-cell lymphoma (EATL) is a term proposed by [20] to describe the rare form of high-grade non-Hodgkin T-cell lymphoma of the upper small intestine associated with CD. Subsequently, in 1989, Holmes and colleagues pointed out that celiac patients have a high risk of developing malignancy, particularly lymphoma. That is corroborated by the findings of studies such as the one from Green et al. [11] and Silano and colleagues (2007), where the most common malignancy identified was non-Hodgkin lymphoma. In this context, Silano et al. [13] conducted another study with a different cohort to evaluate whether strict adherence to the GFD would reduce the risk of developing EATL [13].

The study sample consisted of 1757 patients diagnosed with CD between January 1982 and December 2006. Information about adherence to the GFD was obtained through interviews. Participants were classified into four groups according to the degree of gluten exposure reported in the interview. The first group comprised of patients who strictly followed the GFD; the second group was composed of patients who consumed up to four gluten-containing meals per month; the third group consumed five to ten gluten-containing meals per month; and the fourth group consumed more than 10 gluten-containing meals per month. Most patients (n = 1113) reported complete adherence to the GFD, belonging to the first group (63.4%); 16.9% were classified in the second group (n = 296); 9.8% in the third group (n = 172) and 9.9% in the fourth group (n = 173) [13].

A total of nine patients developed LTAE while the expected number, according to the RMP, was only 1.4. Among these individuals, only four followed a strict GFD after the diagnosis of CD. The authors mentioned that the risk of developing intestinal lymphoma is related to the presence of gluten in the diet, regardless of the number of gluten-containing meals:

> *"It is likely that the chronic stimulation of T-cells in celiac small-bowel mucosa, one of the mechanisms that are supposed to lead to the development of lymphoma, is induced even by a small amount of gluten, and therefore a few monthly dietary indiscretions are sufficient to induce the carcinogenic stimulation."*

This raises concerns about the possibility of patients withholding information during a consultation due to fear of admitting that they are not following the doctor's or other healthcare professional's advice. Omitting just one meal containing gluten per month, for example, may be harmful to the patient in a situation like this. In conclusion, the study pointed out that strict adherence to a GFD is protective against the development of gastrointestinal lymphoma. The authors highlight that individuals with CD should be adequately educated on the importance of complying with a GFD to prevent the appearance of this neoplasia [13].

In 2009, Tursi and colleagues investigated a different aspect from what had been evaluated in the previous studies mentioned above. The researchers explored the manifestation forms of CD (classic, subclinical and silent CD) while evaluating the incidence of malignant and non-malignant complications in a cohort of celiac patients on a GFD. The authors also assessed whether the occurrence of complications was related to non-adherence to the diet. The definitions used for the classification of CD were those of Green and Cellier [21], which state that classic CD is characterized by the presence of gluten-sensitive enteropathy with gastrointestinal symptoms (abdominal pain, diarrhea, weight loss and malabsorption syndrome). Subclinical CD refers to the presence of gluten-sensitive enteropathy with extraintestinal symptoms (iron-deficiency anemia, alopecia, recurrent abortion, among others) and the absence of gastrointestinal symptoms. The silent form of CD refers to the presence of gluten-sensitive enteropathy without any symptoms identified through screening of high-risk groups (first-degree relatives of celiac individuals, patients with insulin-dependent diabetes, down syndrome and thyroid disorders) [14].

The sample consisted of 549 Italian patients with CD, included between 1993 and 2006. Adherence to the GFD was evaluated according to an arbitrary quantitative scale based on the patient's interview, considering whether there were: no food transgressions, less than one food transgression per month or more than one food transgression per month since the time of diagnosis. Regarding the form of CD manifestation, 251 patients (45.72%) presented the classic form of the disease, 262 (47.72%) the subclinical form and 36 (6.56%) the silent form. Regarding compliance to GFD, 381 patients (69.4%) were fully compliant, 112 patients (20.40%) reported less than one food transgression per month, and 56 patients (10.20%) reported at least one food transgression per month [14].

Eighteen patients developed complications while on a GFD, with 14 of them diagnosed with classical CD (77.7%) and four with subclinical CD (22.22%). None of the patients with silent CD presented complications. The most registered complications were neoplasms, observed in seven patients (38.89%). Unlike the findings of the previously mentioned studies, the most common malignancy was not EATL, but rather adenocarcinoma of the small intestine with three cases (n = 3), followed by EATL with two cases (n = 2) and colon carcinoma and mucosa-associated lymphoid tissue (MALT) lymphoma, both with one case each (n = 1). Among individuals with malignancies, six had classical CD, and only one had subclinical CD [14].

Regarding the GFD in patients who developed some type of cancer, results showed that three were compliant with the dietary treatment of CD, while four were not. The authors suggest that adherence to the diet does not seem to be a strong risk factor in the development of complications in celiac patients. Instead, the form of CD manifestation at the time of diagnosis appears to be more important in determining complications, such as in the case of classical CD, where the risk of severe endoscopic and histological damage is higher than in the subclinical and silent forms [14].

In Sweden, Olén et al. [15] also investigated CD characteristics and GFD compliance in regards to the risk of lymphoma. In this case-control study, 59 individuals with CD and lymphoma were identified as cases, and 137 controls which had only a CD diagnosis were matched from a population cohort of 11,650 patients. The degree of adherence to the GFD was evaluated through recorded information (by the patient's nutritionist or physician from CD diagnosis until the end of follow-up) available in the medical records. The degree of GFD compliance was defined as: (i) good compliance (strict adherence to the GFD); (ii) low compliance (occasional exceptions or when the patient did not comply to the GFD) and (iii) compliance unknown (medical records did not contain or had scarce information about the patient's diet) [15].

About 59% of the patients were female (n = 115), and the median age at CD diagnosis was 61 years. There was only one case of Hodgkin lymphoma, while 58 cases of non-Hodgkin lymphoma (NHL). Among the NHL cases, 57% were T-cell type (n = 33), 28% were B-cell type (n = 16), and 15% were unspecified NHL (n = 9). Regarding the location of both Hodgkin lymphoma and NHL, 51% (n = 30) were intestinal, and 42% (n = 27) were extraintestinal. Concerning the degree of compliance with the GFD, 34 (58%) patients in the case group had good compliance, 16 (27%) had poor compliance, and 9 (15%) had compliance unknown. Among the control group patients, 92 (67%) had good compliance, 27 (20%) had poor compliance, and 18 (13%) had compliance unknown [15].

No statistically significant risk of lymphoma in general was found in patients with poor compliance with the GFD. However, individuals with a history of weight loss at the time of CD diagnosis had an increased risk of lymphoma years after this diagnosis. The authors suggest that this may indicate that patients with more severe CD and more pronounced inflammation resulting in weight loss have a higher risk of developing lymphoma [15].

In 2011, Volta, Vicentini and Silano [16] conducted a prospective analysis of the risk of papillary thyroid carcinoma in celiac patients. The study sample included all individuals with CD diagnosed at the Collaborating Centers of the Italian Registry of Celiac Disease between January 1982 and December 2006. A validated form was completed for each patient including demographic data, possible occurrence of thyroid disease and adherence to the GFD. Dietary exposure to gluten was expressed in numerical values from 1 to 4 as follows: "1" for patients who did not consume meals containing gluten, "2" for patients who consumed up to 4 meals containing gluten per month, "3" for patients who consumed 5 to 10 meals containing gluten per month, and "4" for patients who consumed more than 10 meals containing gluten per month [16].

Among the 1757 participants, most were women (n = 1314, 74.7%). The mean age at CD diagnosis was 38.6 ± 12.6 years. A total of six patients were diagnosed with the papillary form of thyroid carcinoma, five of whom were women [16]. The fact that most celiac patients who develop papillary thyroid cancer are female reinforces that both CD and thyroid cancer are more frequent among women [21]. When analyzing the results of this study, it is important to consider that the age at CD diagnosis in patients who developed thyroid carcinoma did not differ statistically from the age of those who did not develop this type of cancer. Moreover, only one patient with carcinoma exhibited poor adherence to the GFD, while the other five had excellent compliance. These findings suggest that early diagnosis of CD and strict adherence to GFD may not confer a protective effect against the development of thyroid malignancy, contrary to what was reported in other studies [16].

In the multicenter retrospective case-control study conducted in four community hospitals in Buenos Aires, Pereyra et al. [17] aimed to determine the risk of colorectal neoplasia among celiac patients by quantifying the prevalence of colorectal polyps, adenomas and advanced neoplastic lesions (ANL) in comparison with healthy patients. Individuals with CD were considered cases, and those without CD were controls. The time since diagnosis and adherence to the GFD were evaluated. To evaluate diet compliance, Biagi's validated questionnaire [22] was used, which is based on four simple questions and provides a final score on five levels (0-IV) that are clinically grouped into three levels: (0) or (I) are individuals who do not follow the GFD; (II) are those who follow the GFD, but with significant errors that require correction; and those with a score of (III) and (VI) follow a strict GFD [17].

During the analyzed period, 118 celiac patients who underwent prior colonoscopy were identified and included in the study as cases, and 236 patients without CD were included as controls. The reason for the colonoscopy was the individual's need to undergo it, which could have been for colorectal cancer (CRC) screening, which is a critical detail in the study. The average age of cases was 56 years. Regarding the GFD compliance of patients with CD, 65% (n = 76) followed a strict GFD (scores III or IV), 20% (n = 23) did not follow a strict GFD (scores 0 or I), and 15% (n = 17) followed a GFD, but with errors that require correction (score II). Concerning the time of CD diagnosis, 41% of patients had been diagnosed for 5 to 10 years (n = 48), 32% had the diagnosis for less than 5 years (n = 37), and 27% had more than 10 years of diagnosis (n = 31). The presence of polyps, adenomas and ANLs in patients with CD was 24 (20%), 18 (15%) and 3 (2.5%), respectively [17].

In this study, the prevalence of colorectal polyps, adenomas and ANLs in celiac patients was not significantly different from that in patients without CD. However, results showed that patients with CD who did not follow a strict GFD had an increased risk for adenomas. Since most patients CD adhered strictly to the GFD, it is uncertain whether the absence of risk for colorectal neoplasia would persist in a larger sample with a higher prevalence of non-adherence to the diet. In conclusion, the authors did not find a higher risk of CRC in patients with CD; however, non-adherence to a strict GFD was an independent predictor for the presence of adenomas [17].

Finally, the Italian study by Volta et al. [18] aimed to describe the risk of colon carcinoma in a group of celiac patients. The study population consisted of patients diagnosed with CD at the Collaborating Centers of the Italian Register for Celiac Disease Complication between January 1982 and December 2006. A total of 1757 patients were included in the study, of whom 74.8% were female (n = 1314), with a mean age of 38.6 years. Information on compliance with the GFD was obtained through interviews, and the sample was divided into four groups according to the monthly frequency of gluten-containing meals. A total of 1113 patients reported adherence to the GFD (63.4%), 296 consumed gluten-containing meals one to four times a month (16.9%), 172 consumed up to 10 gluten-containing meals a month (9.8%), and 173 followed an unrestricted diet (9.9%).

Six patients (four women and two men) developed colon carcinoma during the follow-up period. Among those, four followed the GFD strictly and two did not. The SMR (observed cases = 6; expected cases = 28.9) overall for colon carcinoma was 0.29 (95% CI = 0.07–0.45). The cases for this type of carcinoma observed within 1 year from the diagnosis of CD were incident cases. Therefore, excluding these cases from the analysis to avoid ascertainment bias, the SMR drops to 0.13 (95% CI = 0.03–0.35) [18].

By stratifying the risk according to gluten intake, the SMR decreases even further to 0.07 (95% CI = 0.009–0.27) for CD patients who adhere strictly to the GFD. Furthermore, it is important to mention that all four patients who developed colon carcinoma, despite good adherence to the GFD, were diagnosed with CD at a much older age than the sample in this study (62.8 ± 8.2 vs. 38.6 ± 12.6; $p < 0.05$), which indicates that they maintained a gluten-containing diet for a longer time. In conclusion, the authors suggest that CD patients have a lower risk of developing colon carcinoma compared to the general population. This risk decreases during the first year after CD diagnosis, and it is even lower for treated patients who strictly follow the GFD [18].

4. Conclusion

There is still no consensus in the scientific literature regarding the role of the GFD in the development of malignancies in celiac patients. Some studies suggest that the diet plays a protective role, while others have not found an association between diet and cancer. The most common type of cancer identified in the studies was non-Hodgkin lymphoma, specifically enteropathy-associated T-cell lymphoma, followed by others such as Hodgkin's lymphoma, colon carcinoma, adenocarcinoma of the small intestine and thyroid cancer.

Late CD diagnosis, cancer type and classification of CD form were relevant to the outcomes related to the protective or non-protective role of the GFD. However, it is important to emphasize that the GFD is essential for the clinical, serological and histological recovery of CD patients, also affecting their quality of life, regardless of its effect on the development of neoplasms or not.

This review contributes in pointing out the scarcity of studies that investigated the relation between the GFD and the onset of malignancies in CD and highlights the need to expand research on this topic. In the future, when new articles on the subject are published, the development of a systematic review may provide support for healthcare professionals' recommendations in the prevention of complications associated with CD.

Author details

Maiara Botosso, Renatta Damasceno and Priscila Farage*
Federal University of Goias, Brazil

*Address all correspondence to: priscilafarage@ufg.br

References

[1] Husby S et al. European Society for Pediatric Gastroenterology, Hepatology, and Nutrition guidelines for the diagnosis of coeliac disease. Journal of Pediatric Gastroenterology and Nutrition. 2012;**54**(1):136-160

[2] Bascuñán KA, Vespa MC, Araya M. Celiac disease: Understanding the gluten-free diet. European Journal of Nutrition. 2017;**56**:449-459

[3] Husby S et al. European Society Paediatric Gastroenterology, Hepatology and Nutrition guidelines for diagnosing coeliac disease 2020. Journal of Pediatric Gastroenterology and Nutrition. 2020;**70**(1):141-156

[4] Lebwohl B et al. Association between celiac disease and mortality risk in a Swedish population. Journal of the American Medical Association (JAMA). 2020;**323**(13):1277-1285

[5] Garófolo A et al. Dieta e câncer: Um enfoque epidemiológico. Revista de Nutrição. 2004;**17**(4):491-505

[6] Muscaritoli M et al. ESPEN practical guideline: Clinical nutrition in cancer. Clinical Nutrition. 2021;**40**(5):2898-2913

[7] Ludvigsson JF et al. Small-intestinal histopathology and mortality risk in celiac disease. Journal of the American Medical Association. 2009;**302**(11):1171-1178

[8] Askling J et al. Cancer incidence in a population-based cohort of individuals hospitalized with celiac disease or dermatitis herpetiformis. Gastroenterology. 2002;**123**(5):1428-1435

[9] Makharia GK et al. The global burden of coeliac disease: Opportunities and challenges. Nature Reviews Gastroenterology & Hepatology. 2022;**19**:313-327

[10] Marafini I, Monteleone G, Stolfi C. Association between celiac disease and cancer. International Journal of Molecular Sciences. 2020;**21**(11):4155

[11] Green PH et al. Risk of malignancy in patients with celiac disease. The American Journal of Medicine. 2003;**115**(3):191-195

[12] Silano M et al. Delayed diagnosis of coeliac disease increases cancer risk. BMC Gastroenterology. 2007;7(1):1-5

[13] Silano M et al. Effect of a gluten-free diet on the risk of enteropathy-associated T-cell lymphoma in celiac disease. Digestive Diseases and Sciences. 2007;**53**(4):972-976

[14] Tursi A et al. Complications in celiac disease under gluten-free diet. Digestive Diseases and Sciences. 2009;**54**(10):2175-2182

[15] Olén O et al. Coeliac disease characteristics, compliance to a gluten free diet and risk of lymphoma by subtype. Digestive and Liver Disease. 2011;**43**(11):862-868

[16] Volta U, Vincentini O, Silano M. Papillary cancer of thyroid in celiac disease. Journal of Clinical Gastroenterology. 2011;**45**(5):44-46

[17] Pereyra L et al. Risk of colorectal neoplasia in patients with celiac disease: A multicenter study. Journal of Crohn's and Colitis. 2013;**7**(12):672-677

[18] Volta U et al. Low risk of colon cancer in patients with celiac

disease. Scandinavian Journal of Gastroenterology. 2014;**49**(5):564-568

[19] Holmes GK et al. Malignancy in coeliac disease: Effect of a gluten free diet. Gut. 1989;**30**(3):333-338

[20] O'farrelly CLIONA et al. Humoral response to wheat protein in patients with coeliac disease and enteropathy associated T cell lymphoma. British Medical Journal (Clinical Research Edition). 1986;**293**(6552):908-910

[21] Green PH, Cellier C. Celiac disease. New England Journal of Medicine. 2007;**357**(17):1731-1743

[22] Biagi F et al. A gluten-free diet score to evaluate dietary compliance in patients with coeliac disease. British Journal of Nutrition. 2009;**102**(6):882-887